I0454619

KIDNEY DISEASE

DIET FOR SENIORS ON STAGE 3

COOKBOOK

Healthy and Delicious Low Sodium, Low Potassium, and Low Phosphorus Recipes with Expert Insights for Managing Chronic Kidney Disease

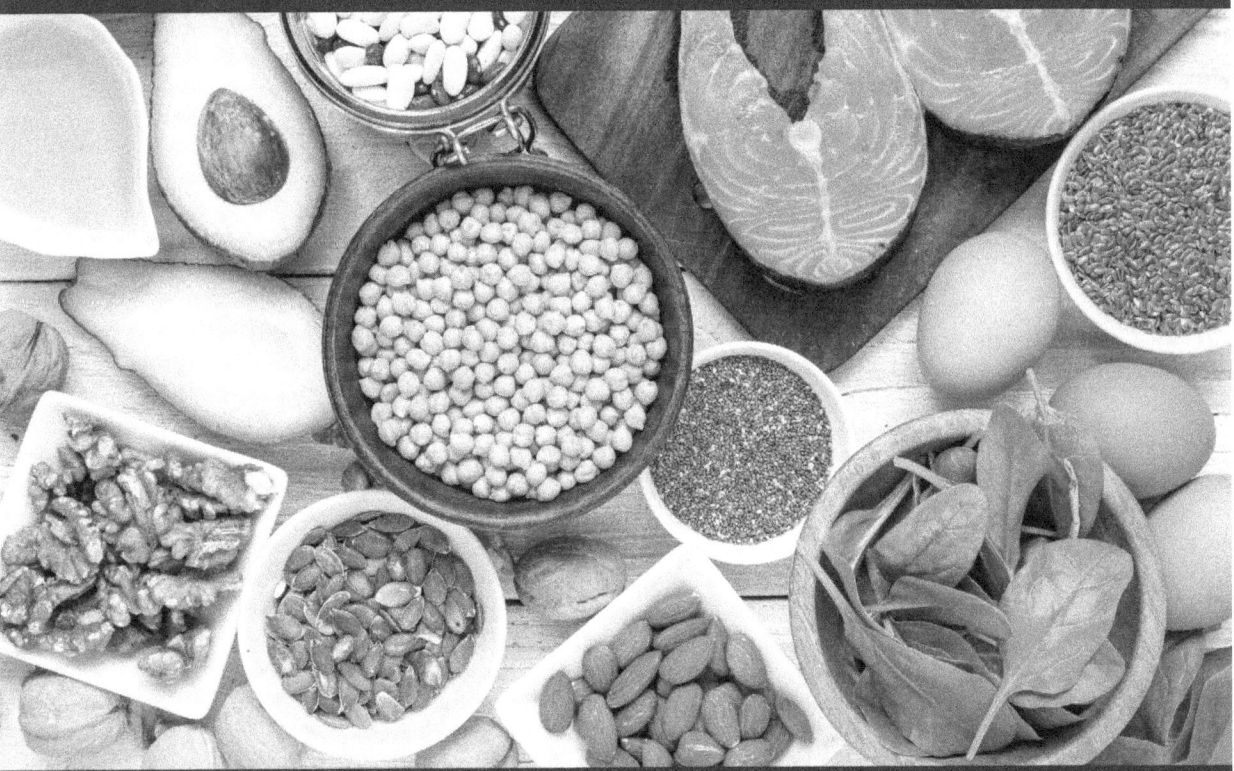

Emily M. Wilson

Copyright © 2023 Dr. Emily M. Wilson

All rights reserved.

No part of this publication may be reproduced, distributed, or transmitted in any form or by any means, including photocopying, recording, or other electronic or mechanical methods, without the prior written permission of the publisher, except in the case of brief quotations embodied in critical reviews and certain other noncommercial uses permitted by copyright law.

Contents

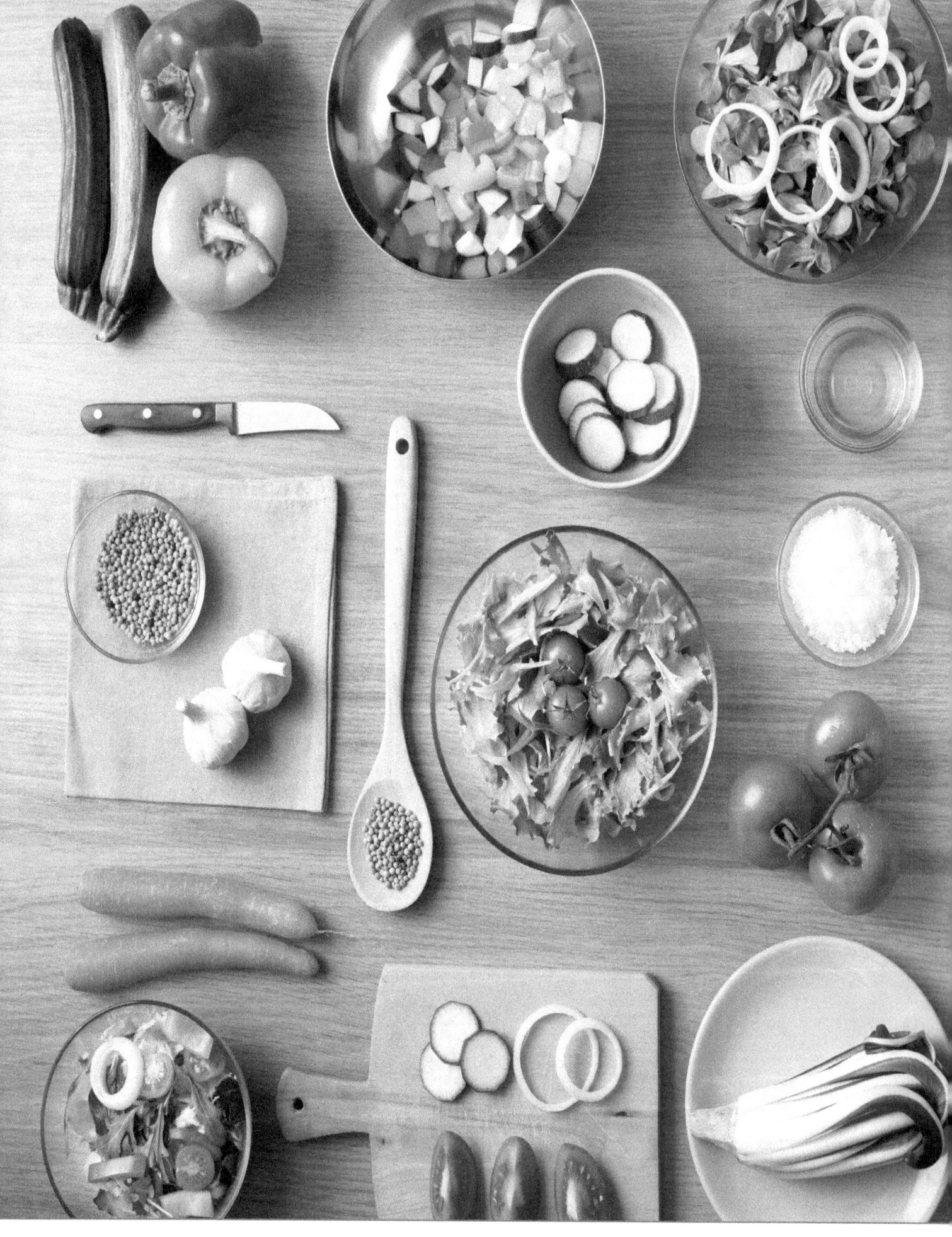

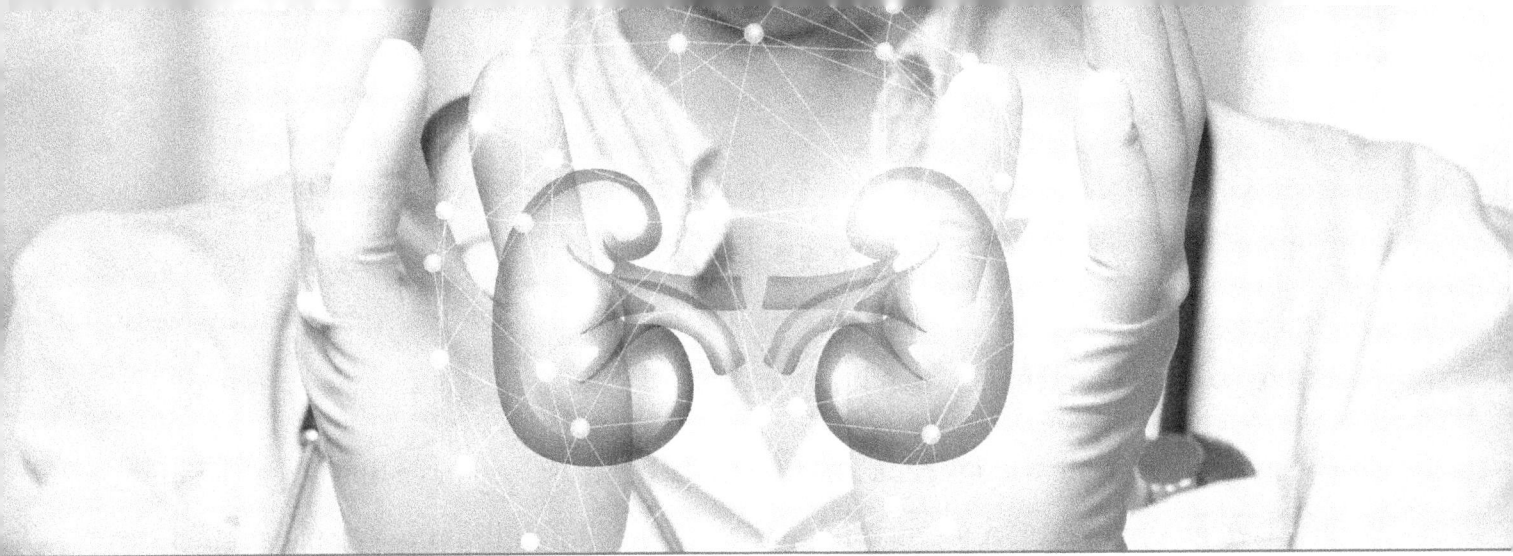

INTRODUCTION

As we age, our bodies undergo various physiological changes, and one of the most critical systems that can be affected is the renal system. Chronic kidney disease (CKD) has emerged as a prevalent health concern among the elderly population, particularly those in stage 3, where the kidneys are moderately impaired. With the increasing prevalence of this condition, it has become imperative to emphasize the vital role of a tailored diet in managing and improving the health outcomes of seniors with stage 3 kidney disease.

According to recent medical data, the incidence of kidney disease in seniors has been on a concerning rise, posing significant challenges to their overall well-being and quality of life. Seniors, due to the natural aging process and possible comorbidities, are more susceptible to the progression of kidney dysfunction. Consequently, this has amplified the importance of implementing a comprehensive dietary approach that addresses the specific nutritional needs and restrictions of individuals in stage 3 kidney disease.

This cookbook serves as a practical and informative guide tailored to meet the dietary requirements and restrictions of seniors with stage 3 kidney disease. It represents a culmination of extensive research and practical experience from the field of nephrology and dietetics, aiming to empower seniors and their caregivers with the necessary knowledge and resources to make informed choices about their diet. The content within this cookbook encapsulates a rich assortment of kidney-friendly recipes, incorporating a diverse array of flavors, textures, and nutrient profiles while strictly adhering to the dietary guidelines essential for managing kidney disease.

By incorporating this cookbook into their daily lives, seniors with stage 3 kidney disease can embark on a journey toward better health and improved management of their condition. With the guidance and knowledge provided within these pages, individuals can make empowered choices, understand the significance of portion control, navigate grocery shopping with ease, and gain valuable insights into the art of mindful dining. This cookbook is not just a collection of recipes; it is a holistic tool for seniors and their caregivers to foster a sense of empowerment and well-being through the powerful medium of nutritious and kidney-friendly cooking.

1.1 Breakfast Recipes

1. Scrambled Egg Whites with Spinach

2. Banana and Almond Butter Pancakes

3. Avocado and Tomato Toast

4. Oatmeal with Fresh Berries

5. Greek Yogurt Parfait

6. Apple-Cinnamon Rice Pudding

7. Spinach and Mushroom Frittata

8. Cinnamon-Spiced Rice Cakes

9. Cottage Cheese with Pineapple

10. Blueberry-Banana Smoothie

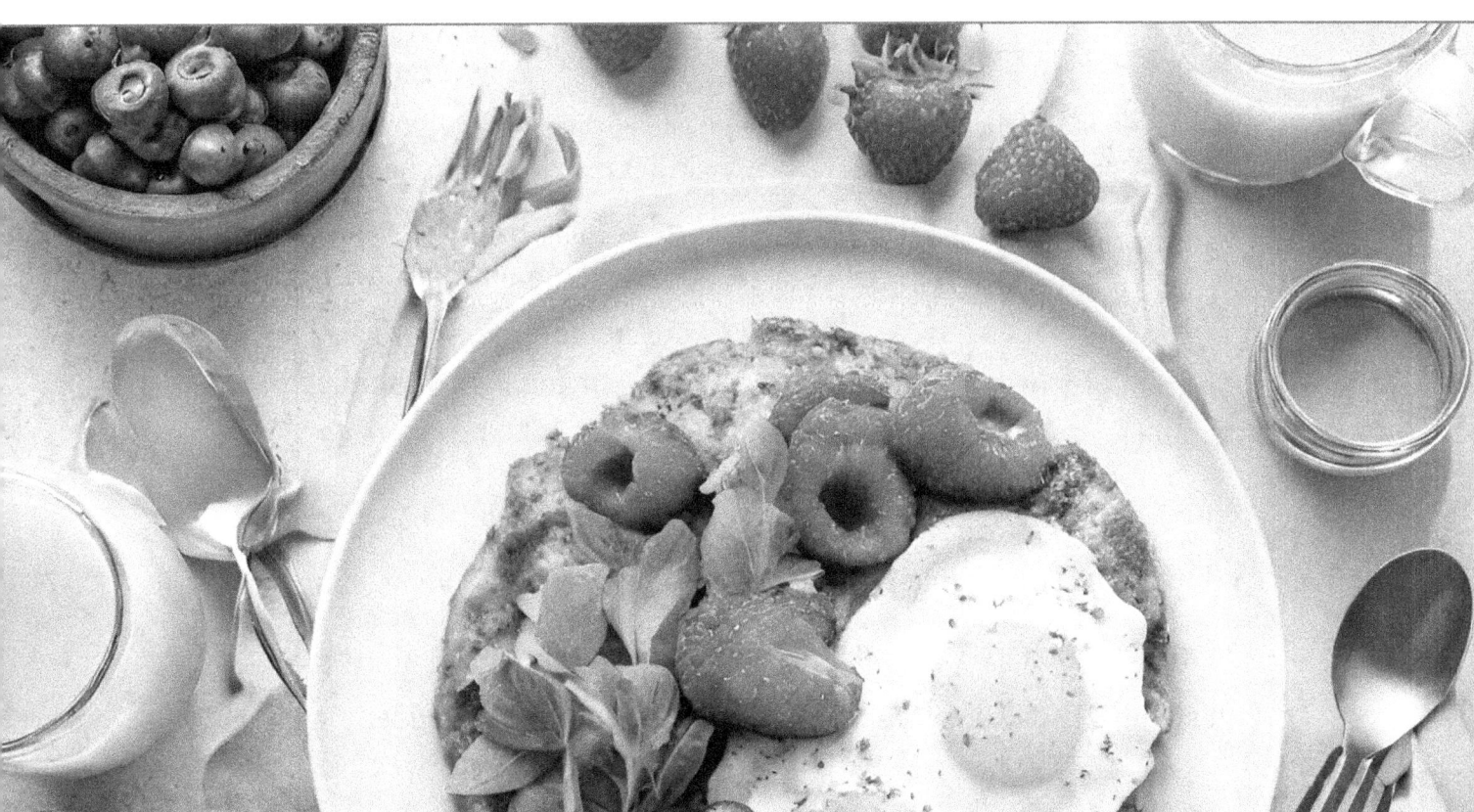

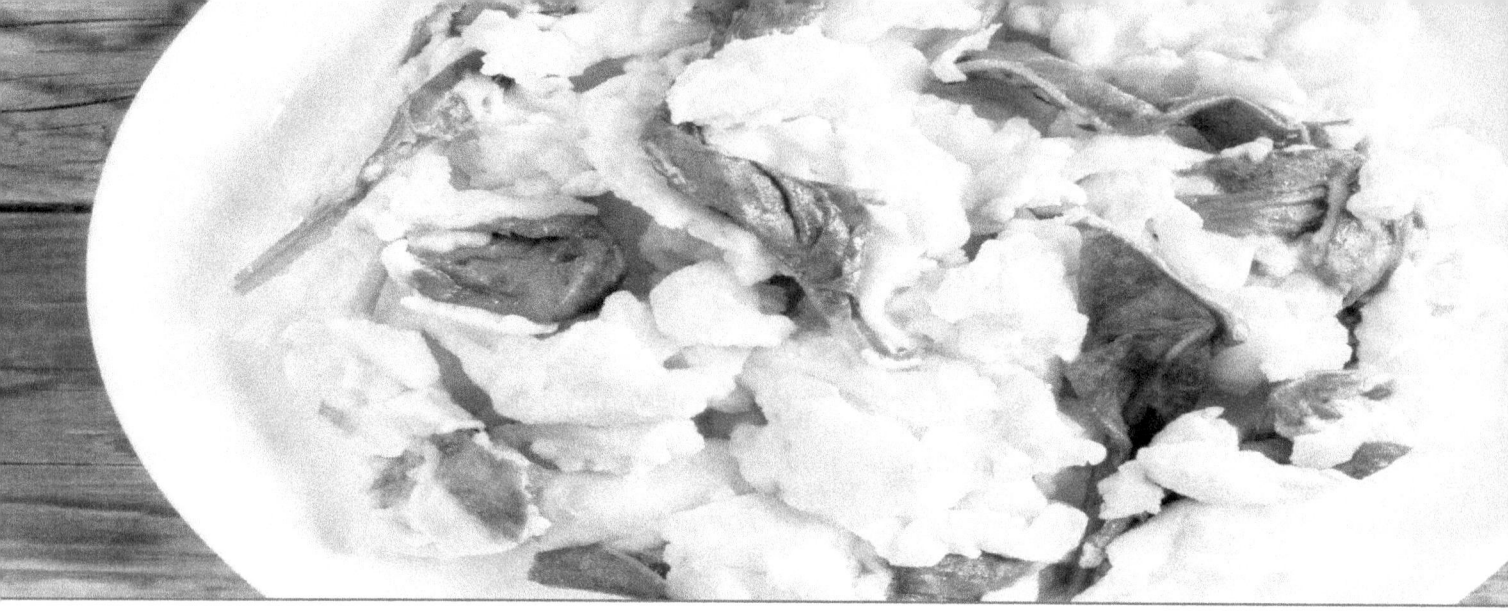

1. Scrambled Egg Whites with Spinach

Benefits: This recipe is high in protein, low in phosphorus, and offers a boost of antioxidants from spinach.

Servings: 2

Ingredients:

- 4 egg whites
- 1 cup fresh spinach, chopped
- 1/4 cup low-fat milk (for creaminess)
- Salt and pepper to taste
- 1 tablespoon olive oil (for cooking)

Prep/Cook Time: 15

Cooking Instructions:

1. Whisk egg whites, milk, salt, and pepper in a bowl.
2. Heat olive oil in a non-stick skillet over medium heat.
3. Add chopped spinach and sauté for a few minutes until wilted.
4. Pour in the egg mixture and cook, stirring gently, until eggs are fully cooked.

Nutritional Information (per serving): Approximately 120 calories, 12g protein, 2g carbohydrates, 0g fiber, 1g sugar, 7g fat, 230mg sodium.

Modification Tip: For lower phosphorus, skip the milk and use egg substitutes. You can also add mushrooms or peppers for added flavor and variety.

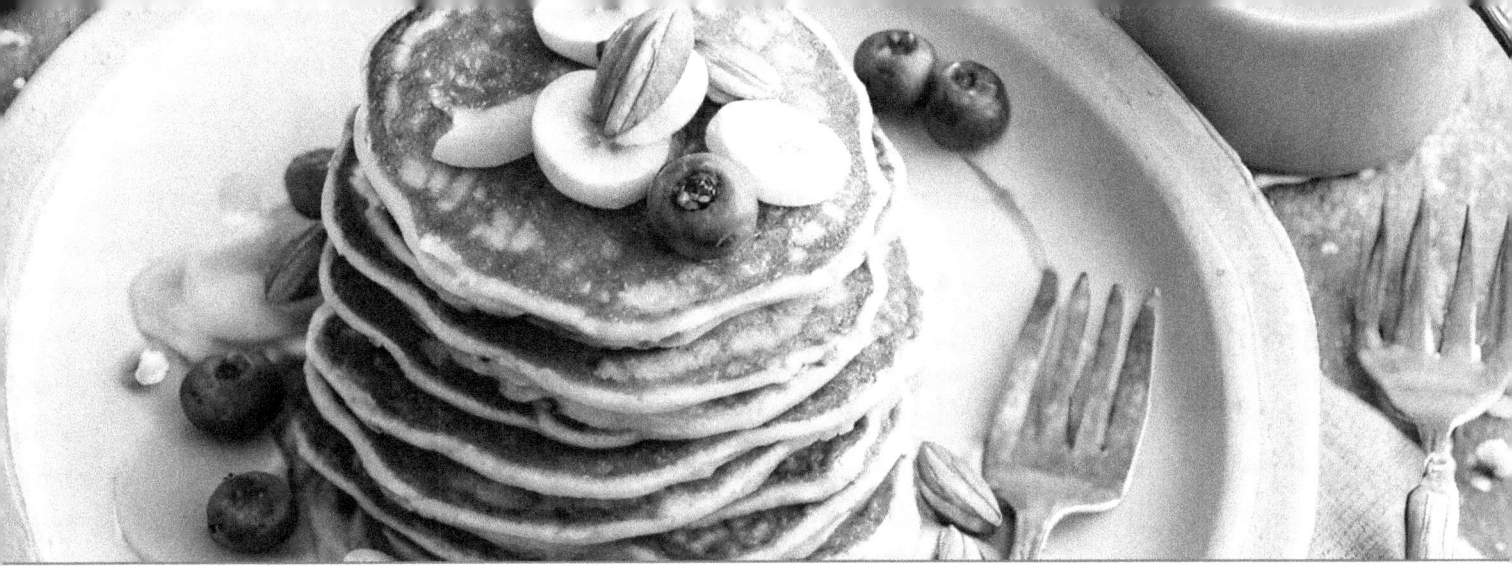

2. Banana and Almond Butter Pancakes

Benefits: This recipe is a delicious way to enjoy a pancake breakfast while keeping potassium in check.

Servings: 2

Prep/Cook Time: 20

Ingredients:

- 1 medium ripe banana
- 2 tablespoons almond butter
- 2 large eggs
- 1/4 teaspoon cinnamon
- Cooking spray (for the pan)

Cooking Instructions:

1. Mash the ripe banana in a bowl.
2. Add almond butter, eggs, and cinnamon, and whisk together until smooth.
3. Heat a non-stick skillet over medium heat and lightly coat with cooking spray.
4. Pour pancake batter onto the skillet and cook until bubbles form on the surface, then flip and cook the other side.
5. Serve with a sprinkle of cinnamon.

Nutritional Information (per serving): Approximately 290 calories, 12g protein, 21g carbohydrates, 4g fiber, 9g sugar, 18g fat, 120mg sodium.

Modification Tip: To lower potassium, choose fruits like apple or pear instead of banana. If you're concerned about phosphorus, consider using sunflower seed butter instead of almond butter.

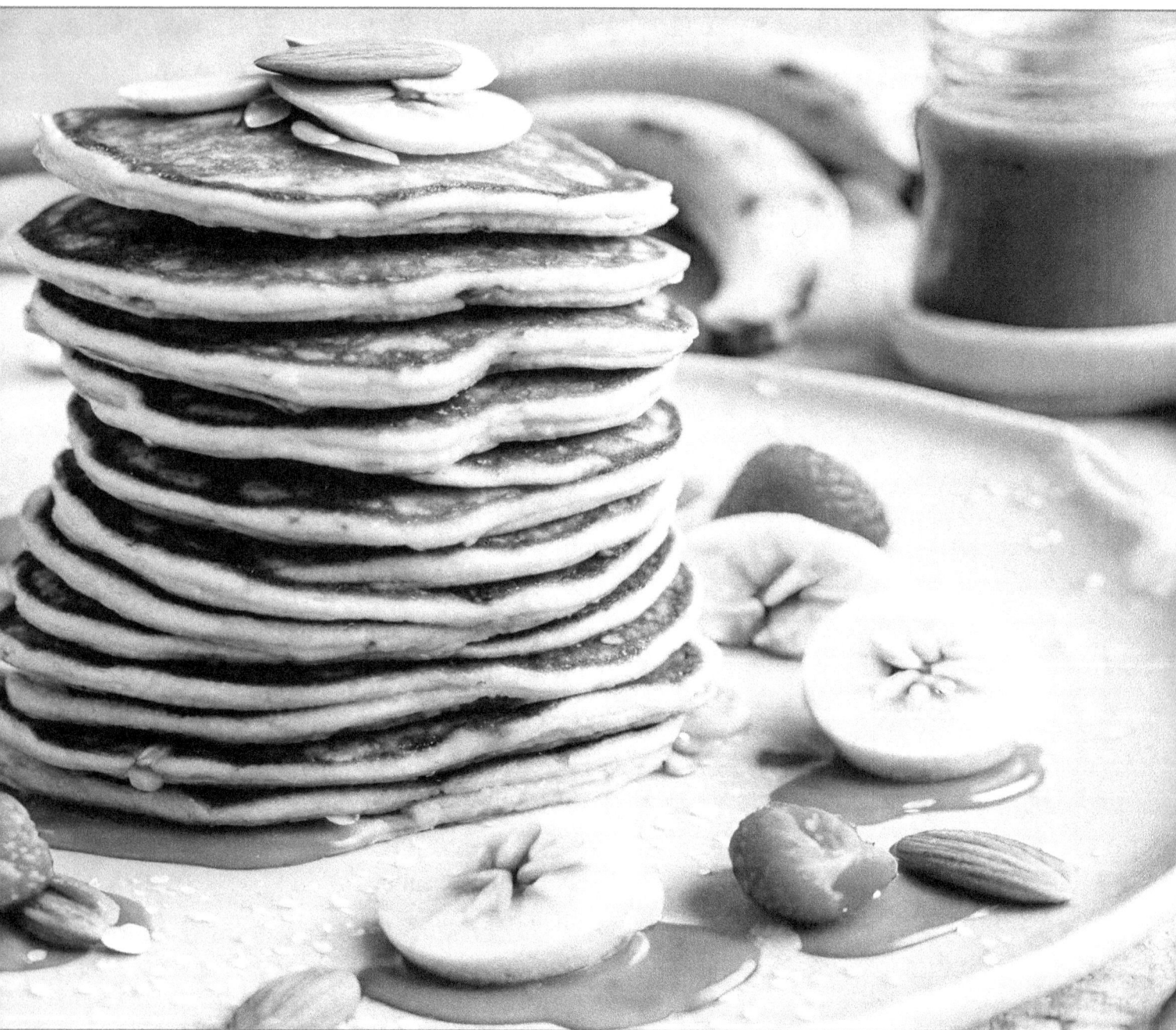

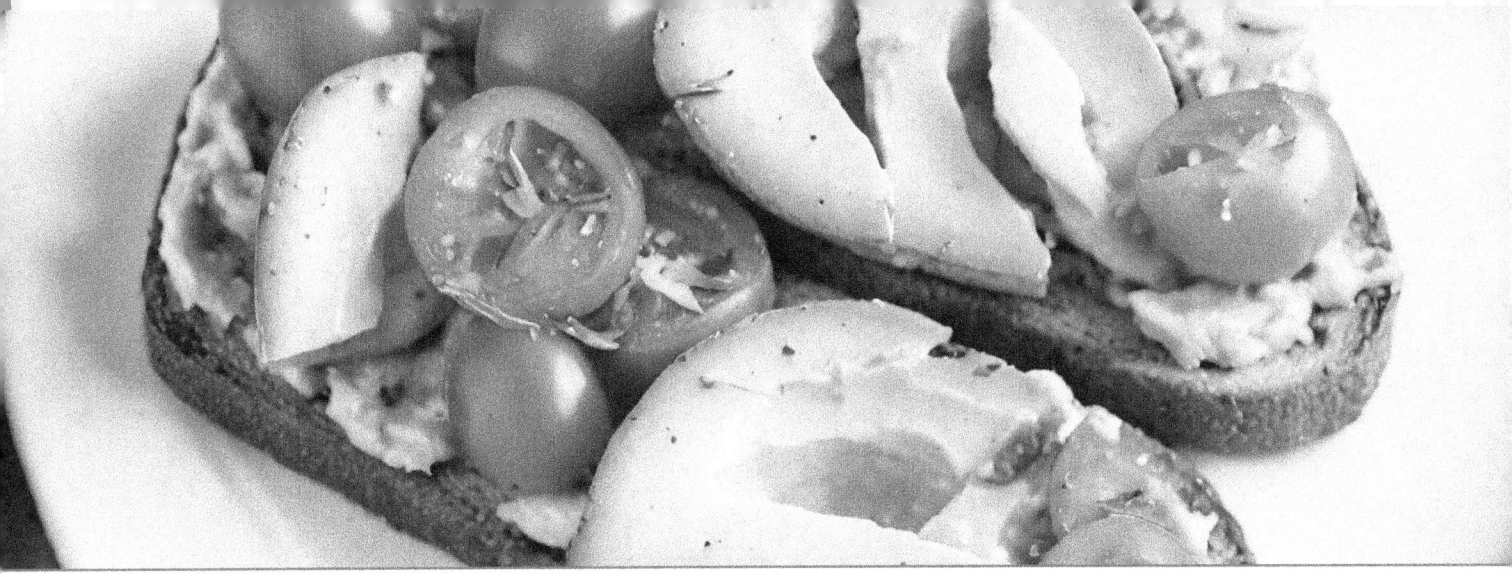

3. Avocado and Tomato Toast

Benefits: Avocado provides healthy fats, while tomatoes offer antioxidants and a burst of flavor.

Servings: 1   Prep/Cook Time: 10

Ingredients:

- 1 slice whole-grain bread
- 1/2 ripe avocado
- 1/2 medium tomato, sliced
- Salt and pepper to taste
- 1 teaspoon olive oil (optional)

Cooking Instructions:

1. Toast the whole-grain bread to your desired level of crispiness.
2. Mash the ripe avocado and spread it onto the toasted bread.
3. Top with tomato slices and season with salt and pepper.
4. For added flavor, drizzle with a touch of olive oil.

Nutritional Information (per serving): Approximately 220 calories, 4g protein, 20g carbohydrates, 6g fiber, 2g sugar, 14g fat, 180mg sodium.

Modification Tip: To reduce sodium, use less salt or omit it. You can also add a dash of lemon juice for extra flavor without sodium.

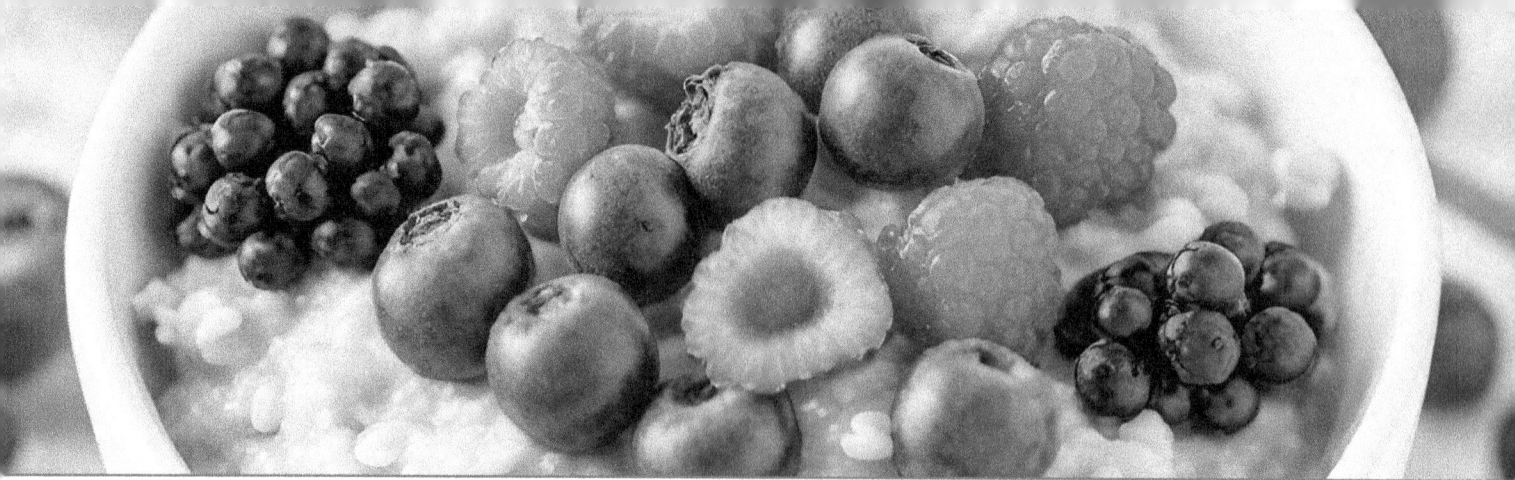

4. Oatmeal with Fresh Berries

Benefits: Oatmeal is a kidney-friendly source of fiber and complex carbohydrates. Berries provide antioxidants and natural sweetness.

Servings: 2

Ingredients:

- 1 cup old-fashioned oats
- 2 cups water
- 1 cup mixed fresh berries (e.g., strawberries, blueberries)
- 1 tablespoon honey (optional)
- 1 tablespoon chopped nuts (e.g., almonds or walnuts)

Prep/Cook Time: 10 Minutes

Cooking Instructions:

1. Boil the water and add oats.
2. Simmer for about 5 minutes or until the oats are cooked and the mixture thickens.
3. Divide into two bowls.
4. Top each with a half-cup of mixed berries.
5. Drizzle honey (if desired) and sprinkle chopped nuts for added flavor.

Nutritional Information (per serving): Approximately 260 calories, 7g protein, 48g carbohydrates, 6g fiber, 5g sugar, 5g fat, 0mg sodium.

Modification Tip: If berries are too high in potassium, consider using apples or pears for a lower potassium alternative.

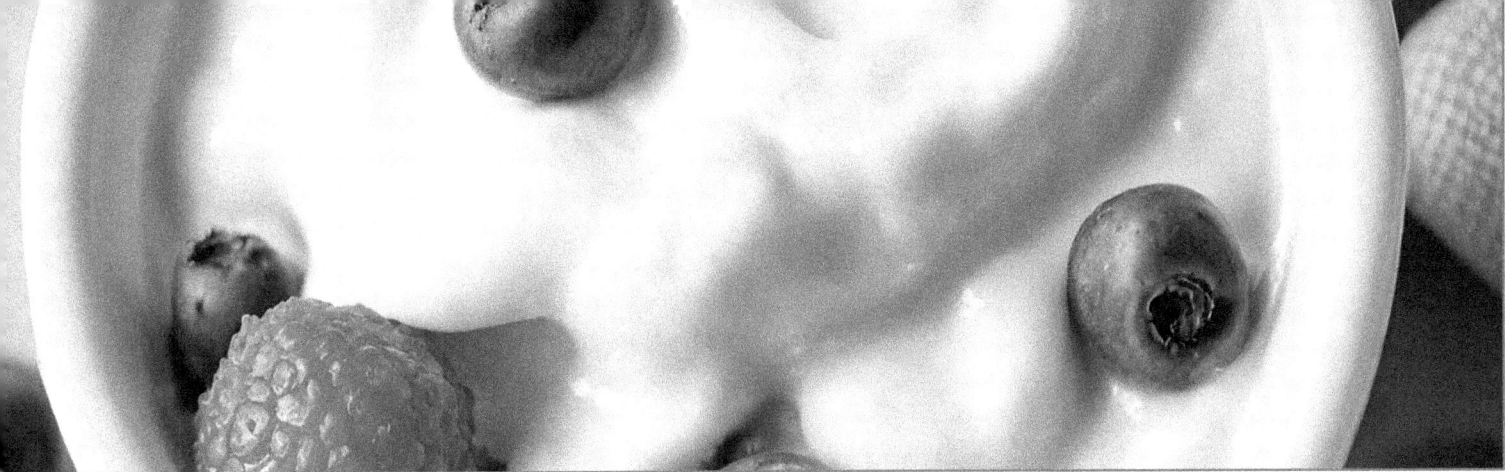

5. Greek Yogurt Parfait

Benefits: Greek yogurt is high in protein, and this recipe provides essential probiotics, fiber, and antioxidants from fruits and nuts.

Servings: 1

Ingredients:

- 1 cup low-fat Greek yogurt
- 1/2 cup mixed fresh berries
- 1 tablespoon chopped almonds
- 1 teaspoon honey (optional)

Prep/Cook Time: 5 Minutes

Cooking Instructions:

1. In a glass or bowl, layer Greek yogurt, fresh berries, and chopped almonds.
2. Drizzle with honey for added sweetness if desired.

Nutritional Information (per serving): Approximately 300 calories, 20g protein, 30g carbohydrates, 4g fiber, 19g sugar, 12g fat, 60mg sodium.

Modification Tip: If you need to reduce potassium, opt for berries with lower potassium content, like raspberries or cranberries. You can also use crushed graham crackers instead of nuts.

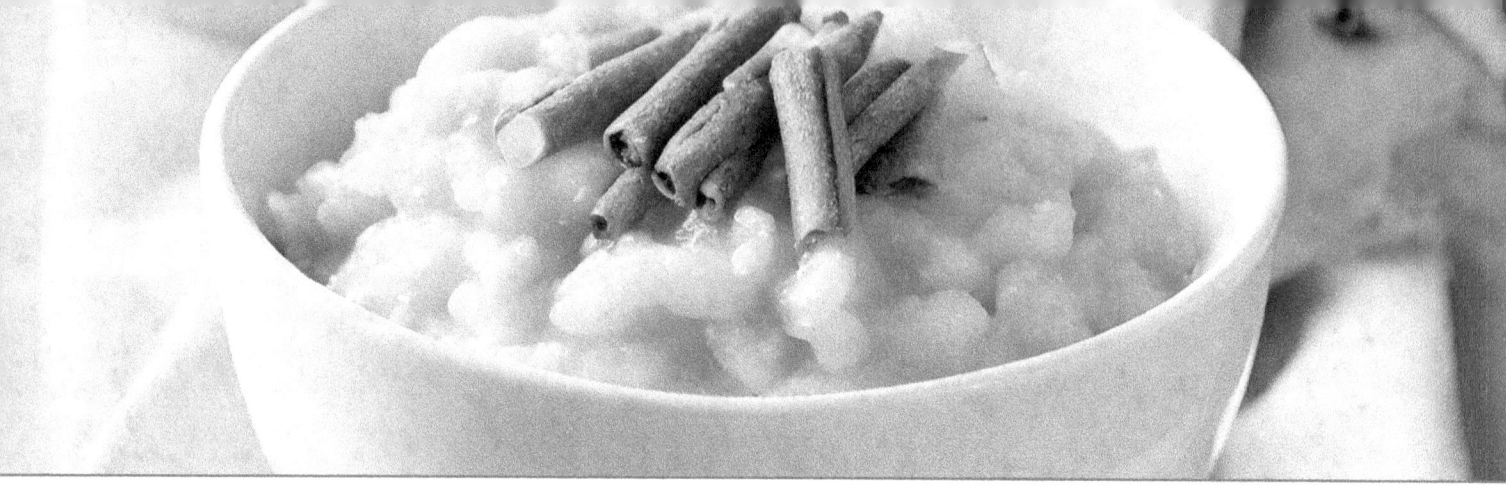

6. Apple-Cinnamon Rice Pudding

Benefits: Rice pudding offers a comforting and low-protein breakfast option for kidney patients.

Servings: 2

Ingredients:

- 1/2 cup Arborio rice
- 2 cups low-fat milk
- 1/2 cup unsweetened applesauce
- 1/2 teaspoon ground cinnamon
- 2 teaspoons sugar or sugar substitute (optional)

Prep/Cook Time: 20 Minutes

Cooking Instructions:

1. In a saucepan, combine rice, milk, applesauce, and cinnamon.
2. Cook over low heat, stirring frequently until the mixture thickens and the rice is tender (about 15-20 minutes).
3. Sweeten with sugar or sugar substitute, if desired.

Nutritional Information (per serving): Approximately 250 calories, 8g protein, 51g carbohydrates, 1g fiber, 15g sugar, 2g fat, 100mg sodium.

Modification Tip: If potassium is a concern, reduce the amount of applesauce or choose a lower potassium fruit. You can also skip the sugar or use a sugar substitute to reduce sugar content.

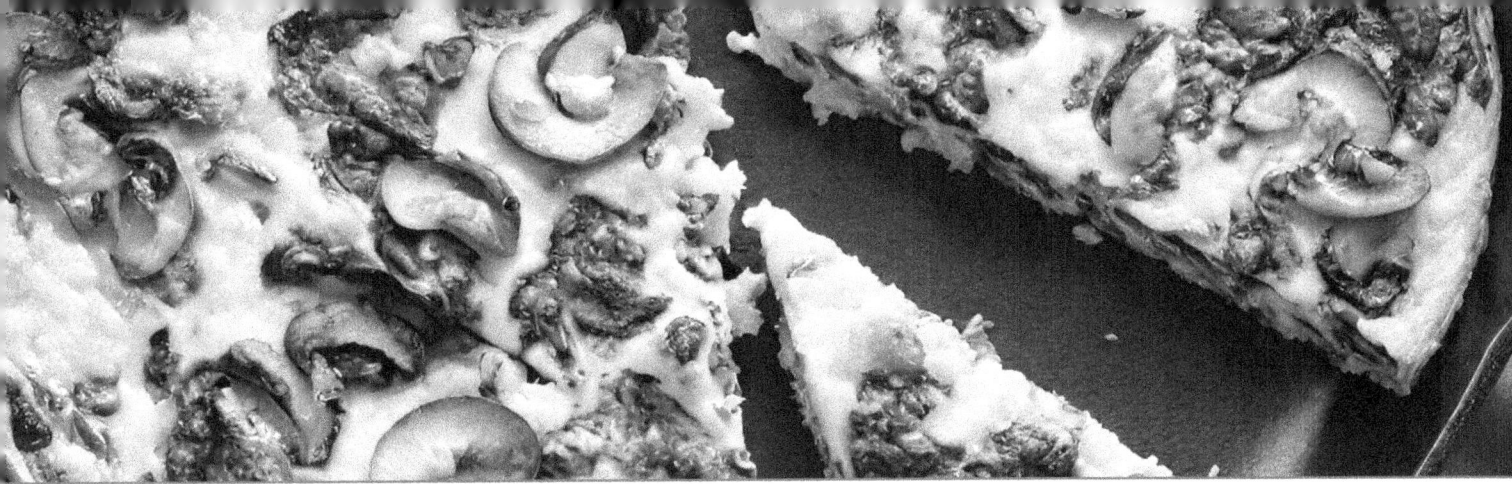

7. Spinach and Mushroom Frittata

Benefits: This frittata is packed with protein, low in phosphorus, and provides a dose of vitamins and minerals.

Servings: 4

Ingredients:

- 8 large egg whites
- 1 cup fresh spinach, chopped
- 1 cup mushrooms, sliced
- 1/4 cup low-fat milk
- Salt and pepper to taste
- 1 tablespoon olive oil (for cooking)

Prep/Cook Time: 30 Minutes

Cooking Instructions:

1. Preheat the oven to 350°F (175°C).
2. In a bowl, whisk egg whites, milk, salt, and pepper.
3. Heat olive oil in an ovenproof skillet over medium heat.
4. Add chopped spinach and sliced mushrooms; sauté for a few minutes until they soften.
5. Pour the egg mixture over the veggies.
6. Place the skillet in the oven and bake for about 15-20 minutes, or until the frittata is set.

Nutritional Information (per serving): Approximately 70 calories, 10g protein, 2g carbohydrates, 1g fiber, 1g sugar, 2g fat, 60mg sodium.

Modification Tip: For lower potassium, choose different vegetables like zucchini or bell peppers. You can also use egg substitutes to reduce phosphorus.

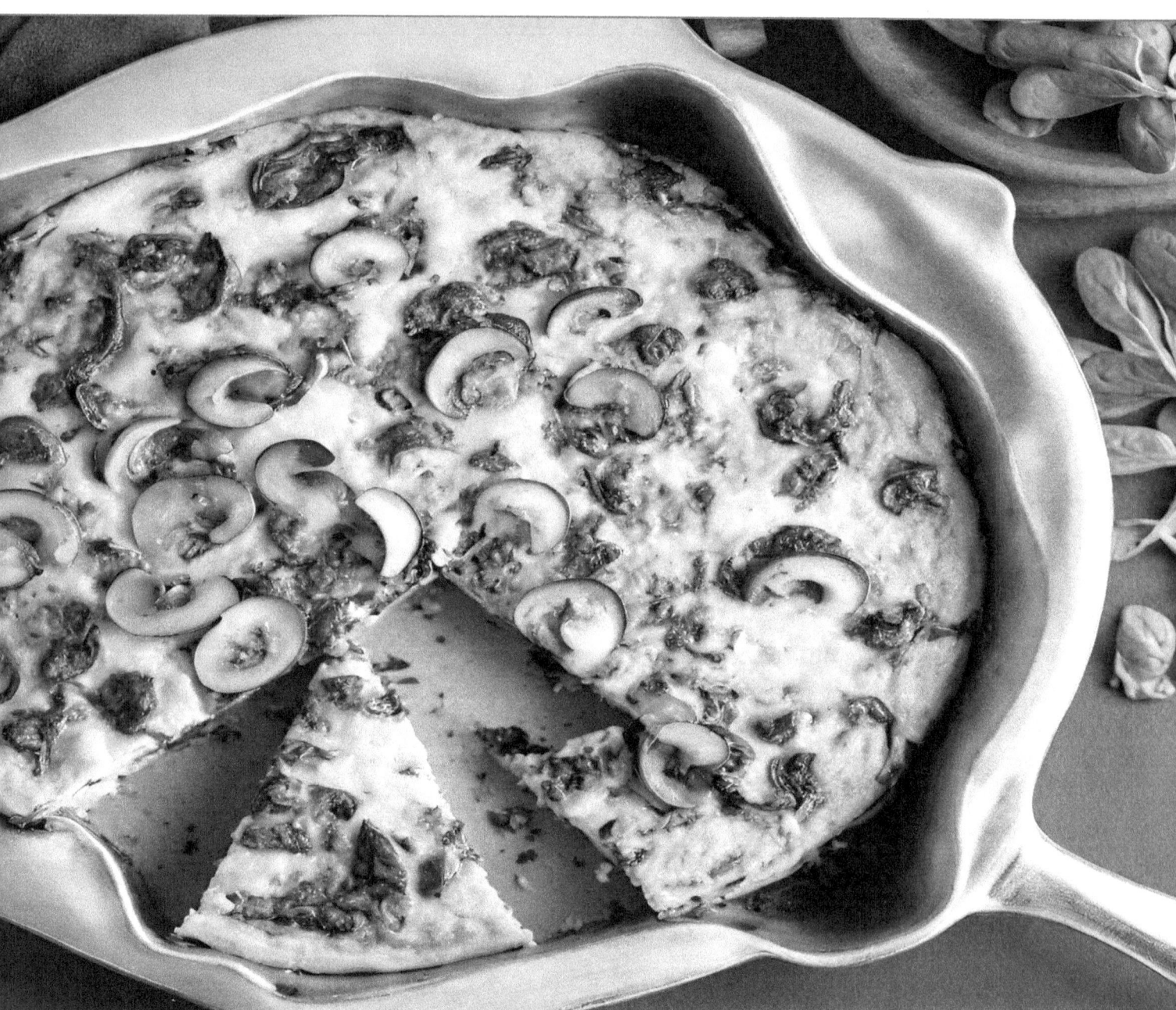

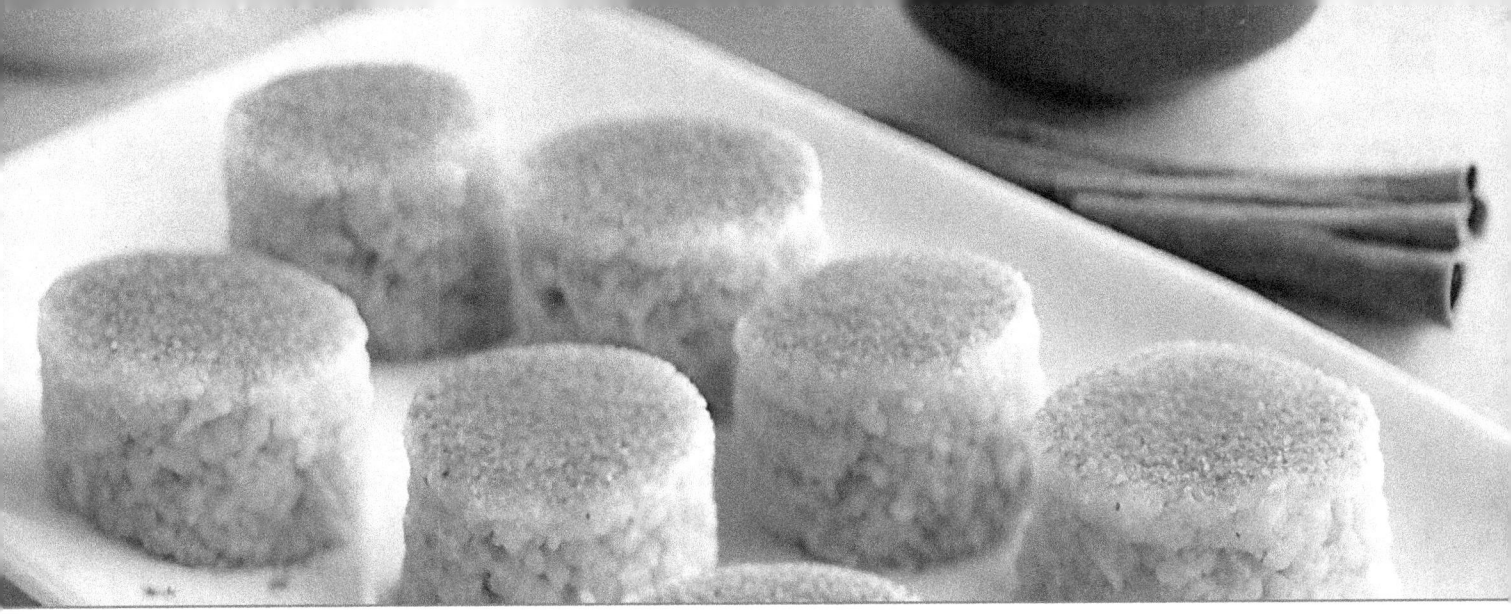

8. Cinnamon-Spiced Rice Cakes

Benefits: Rice cakes provide a low-protein and low-phosphorus base, while cinnamon adds flavor and may help regulate blood sugar.

Servings: 2

Ingredients:

- 2 rice cakes (low-sodium)
- 1/2 teaspoon ground cinnamon
- 1 tablespoon unsalted almond butter.

Prep/Cook Time: 5 Minutes

Cooking Instructions:

1. Spread almond butter on the rice cakes.
2. Sprinkle ground cinnamon on top for added flavor.

Nutritional Information (per serving): Approximately 100 calories, 3g protein, 12g carbohydrates, 1g fiber, 0g sugar, 4g fat, 0mg sodium.

Modification Tip: Ensure you choose low-sodium rice cakes, and consider using sunflower seed butter for a lower phosphorus alternative.

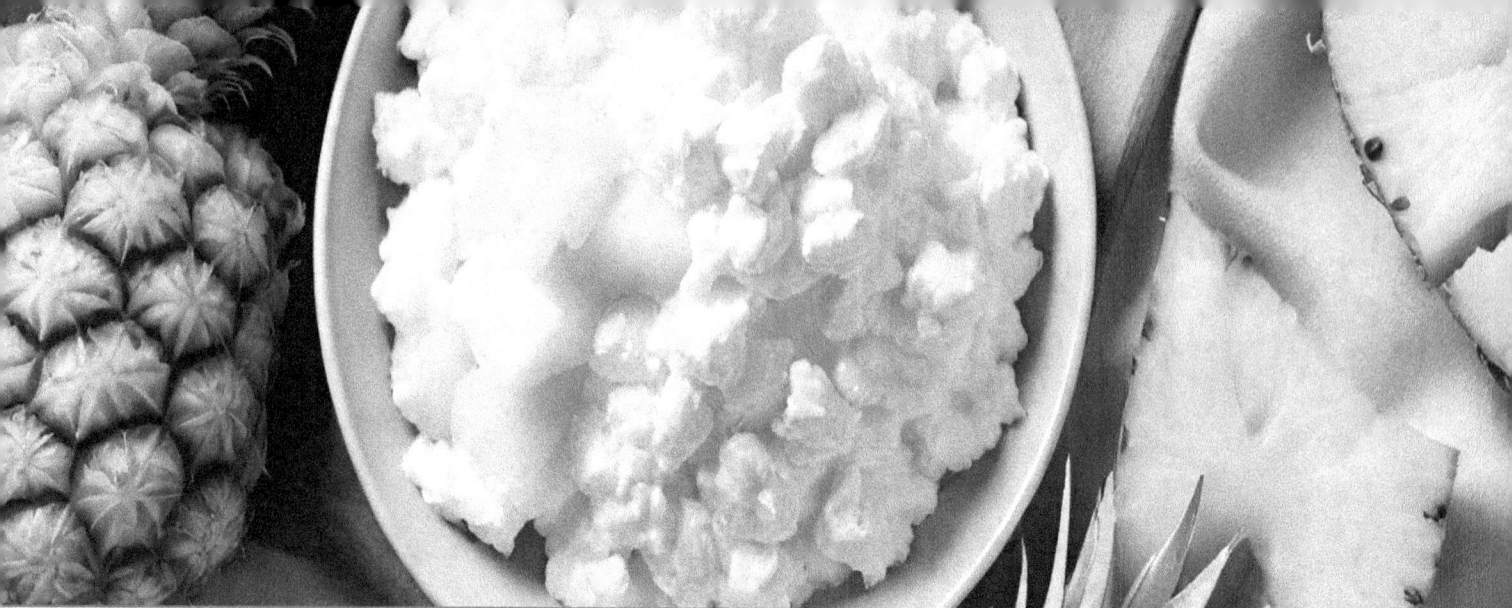

9. Cottage Cheese with Pineapple

Benefits: Cottage cheese is a good source of protein, and pineapple adds a tropical twist while offering vitamin C.

Servings: 1

Prep/Cook Time: 5 Minutes

Ingredients:

- 1/2 cup low-fat cottage cheese
- 1/2 cup fresh pineapple, diced

Cooking Instructions:

1. In a bowl, combine cottage cheese and diced pineapple.
2. Stir gently and serve.

Nutritional Information (per serving): Approximately 160 calories, 14g protein, 22g carbohydrates, 1g fiber, 18g sugar, 2g fat, 390mg sodium.

Modification Tip: Opt for lower sodium cottage cheese and consider using fresh melon or berries if pineapple is too high in potassium.

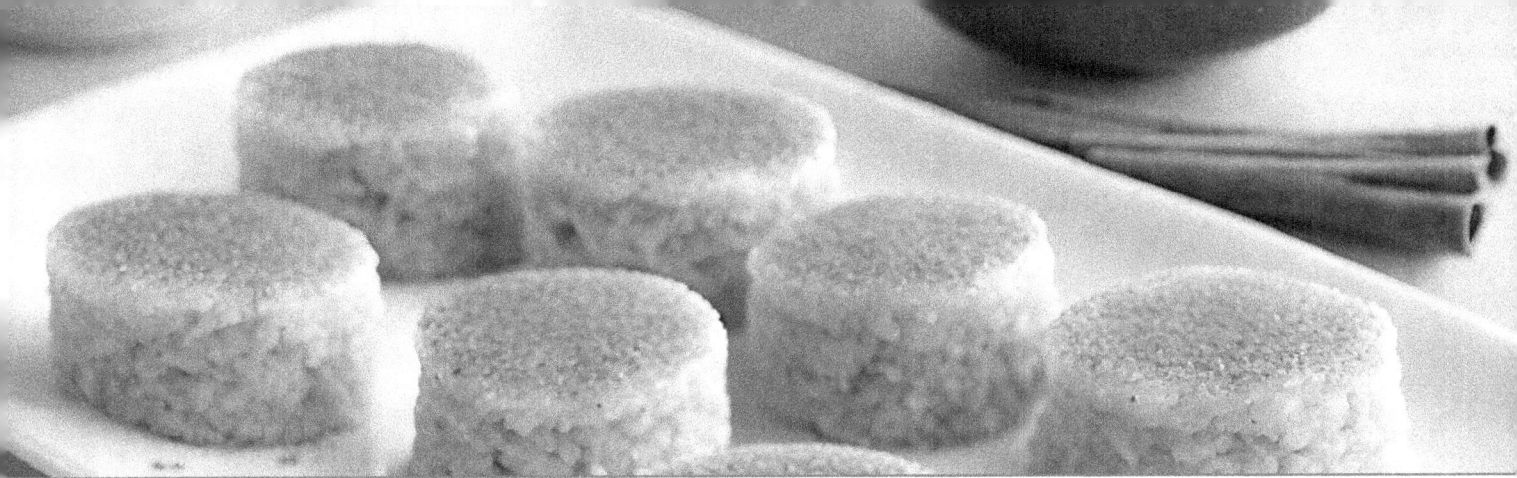

10. Blueberry-Banana Smoothie

Benefits: This smoothie is a quick and convenient way to get protein and antioxidants.

Servings: 1

Ingredients:

- 1/2 cup frozen blueberries
- 1/2 medium banana
- 1/2 cup low-fat yogurt
- 1/2 cup water
- 1 tablespoon honey (optional)

Prep/Cook Time: 5 Minutes

Cooking Instructions:

1. Blend frozen blueberries, banana, yogurt, and water until smooth.

2. Sweeten with honey, if desired.

Nutritional Information (per serving): Approximately 200 calories, 8g protein, 42g carbohydrates, 4g fiber, 27g sugar, 1g fat, 60mg sodium.

Modification Tip: Choose lower potassium fruits such as strawberries or kiwi, and use non-dairy yogurt if needed to reduce phosphorus.

1.2 Lunch Recipes

11. Lemon-Herb Grilled Chicken

12. Quinoa and Vegetable Salad

13. Baked Salmon with Dill

14. Black Bean and Vegetable Soup

15. Turkey and Cranberry Wrap

16. Cucumber and Dill Salad

17. Vegetable Stir-Fry with Tofu

18. Egg Salad with Fresh Herbs

19. Lentil Soup

20. Tuna and White Bean Salad

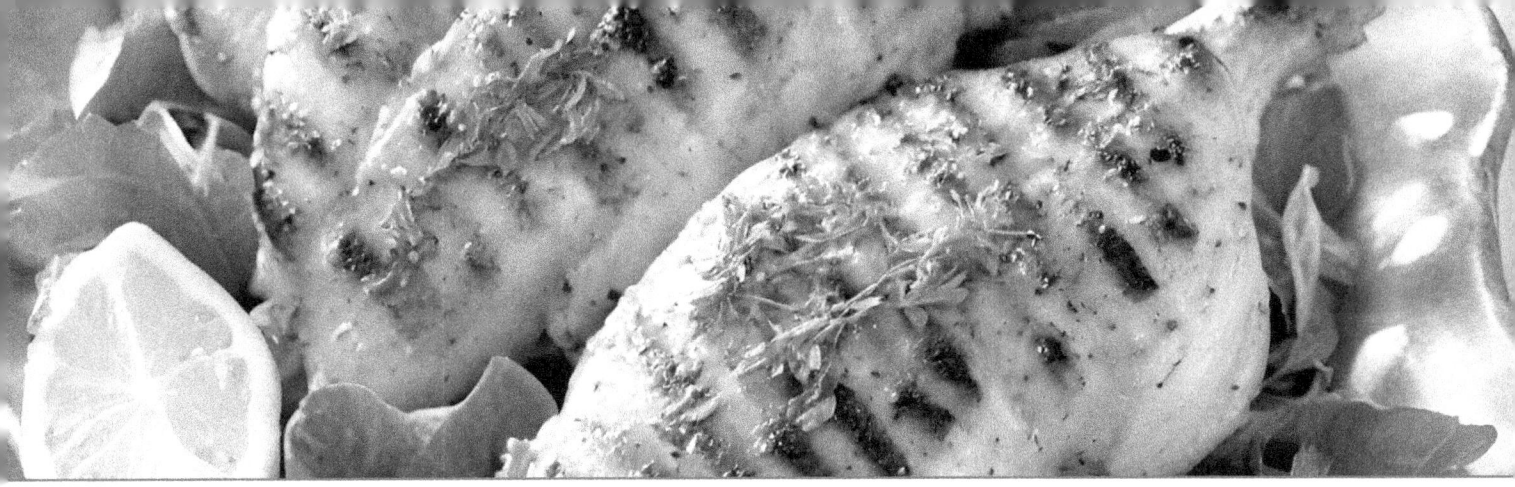

11. Lemon-Herb Grilled Chicken

Benefits: Benefits: This recipe provides lean protein with minimal phosphorus and potassium.

Servings: 2

Ingredients:

- 2 boneless, skinless chicken breasts (4-6 ounces each)
- 1 lemon (juice and zest)
- 1 clove garlic, minced
- 1 tablespoon fresh hcrbs (c.g., rosemary, thyme), chopped
- Salt and pepper to taste
- Olive oil (for grilling)

Prep/Cook Time: 30 Minutes

Cooking Instructions:

1. In a bowl, combine lemon juice, lemon zest, minced garlic, fresh herbs, salt, and pepper.
2. Marinate chicken breasts in this mixture for 20 minutes.
3. Preheat the grill to medium heat and lightly brush it with olive oil.
4. Grill chicken for about 6-8 minutes per side, or until cooked through.

Nutritional Information (per serving): Approximately 180 calories, 26g protein, 2g carbohydrates, 1g fiber, 1g sugar, 7g fat, 70mg sodium.

Modification Tip: For lower phosphorus, consider using a phosphate binder before the meal and reduce the portion size of chicken.

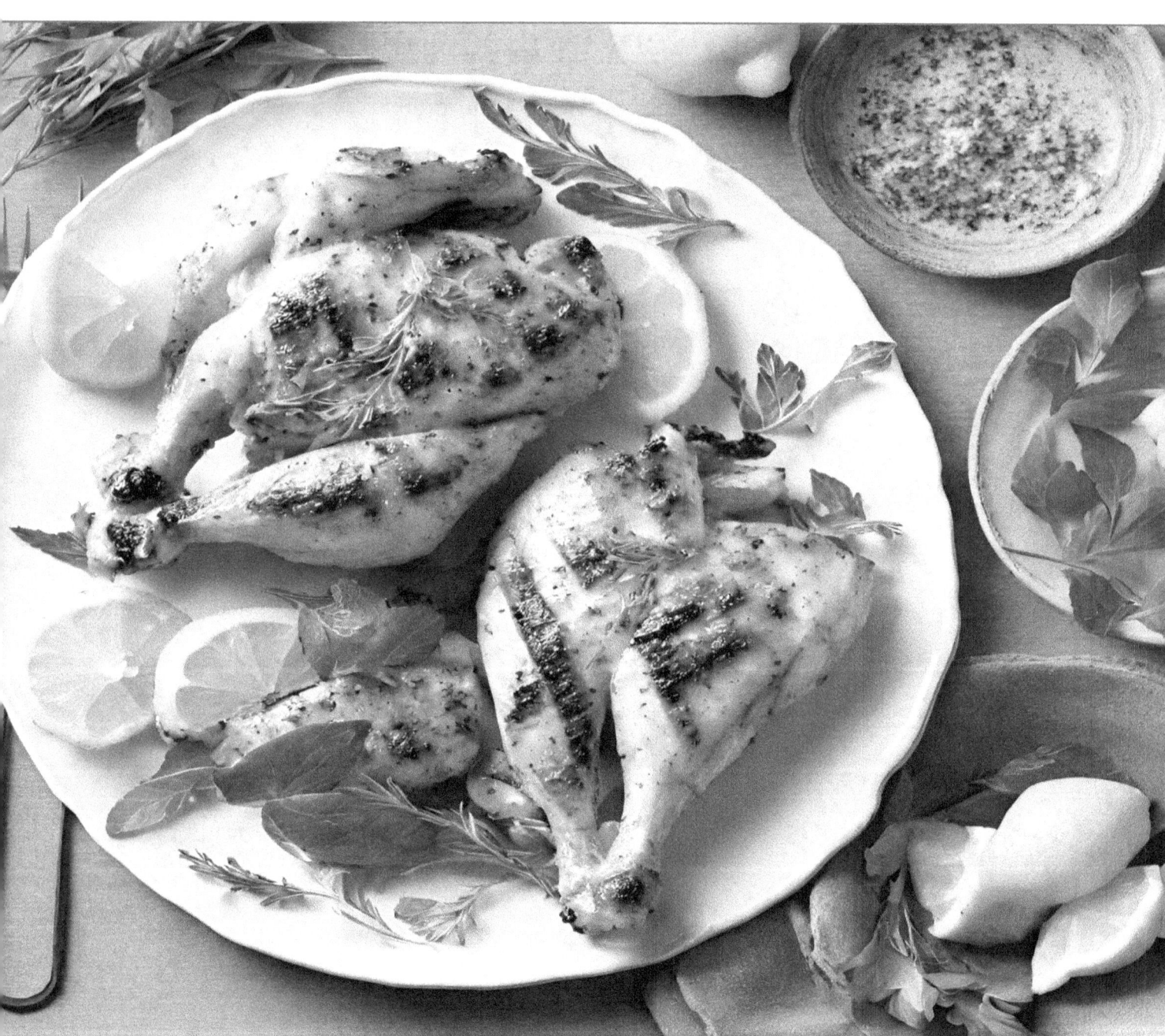

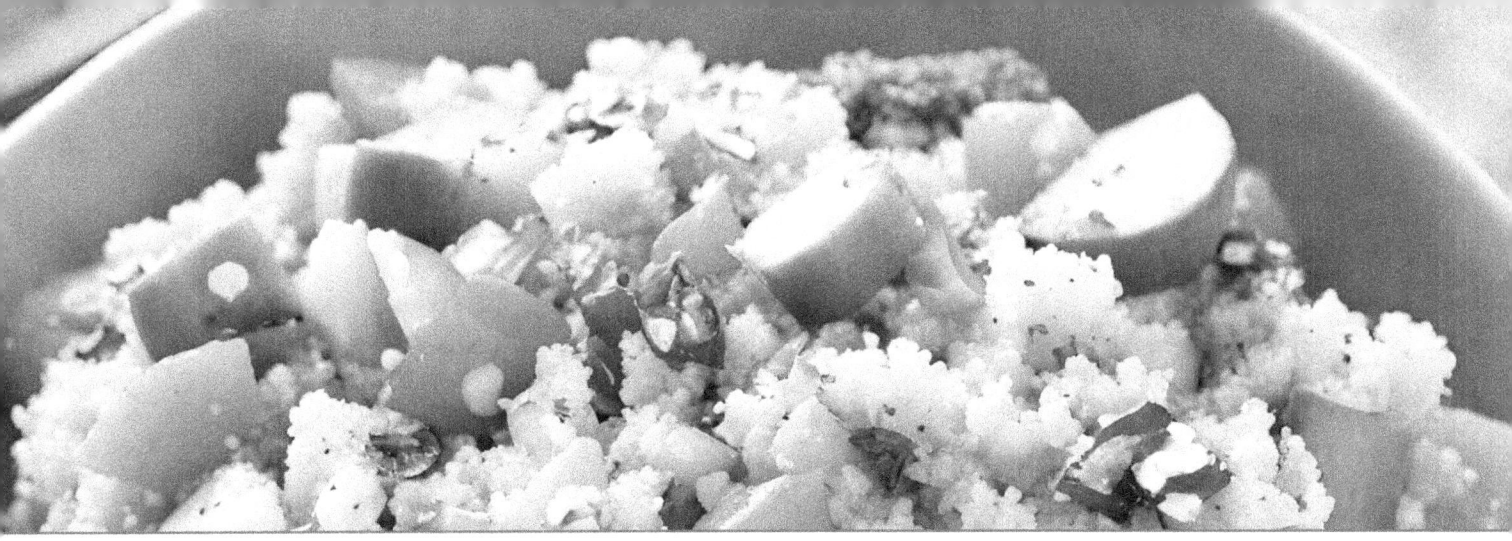

12. Quinoa and Vegetable Salad

Benefits: Quinoa is a high-quality protein source, and this salad offers a variety of essential nutrients and fiber.

Servings: 4

Prep/Cook Time: 25 Minutes

Ingredients:

- 1 cup quinoa, rinsed
- 2 cups water
- 1 cup cucumbers, diced
- 1 cup red bell peppers, diced
- 1/2 cup red onion, finely chopped
- 1/4 cup fresh parsley, chopped
- 1/4 cup olive oil
- 2 tablespoons lemon juice
- Salt and pepper to taste

Cooking Instructions:

1. Boil 2 cups of water and add quinoa. Simmer for about 15 minutes or until quinoa is cooked and water is absorbed.
2. In a large bowl, combine cooked quinoa, cucumbers, red bell peppers, red onion, and fresh parsley.
3. In a separate bowl, whisk together olive oil, lemon juice, salt, and pepper.
4. Drizzle the dressing over the salad and toss to combine.

Nutritional Information (per serving): Approximately 270 calories, 7g protein, 32g carbohydrates, 4g fiber, 3g sugar, 14g fat, 15mg sodium.

Modification Tip: To reduce potassium, opt for a lower-potassium vegetable mix, such as zucchini or green beans. You can also add grilled chicken or tofu for extra protein.

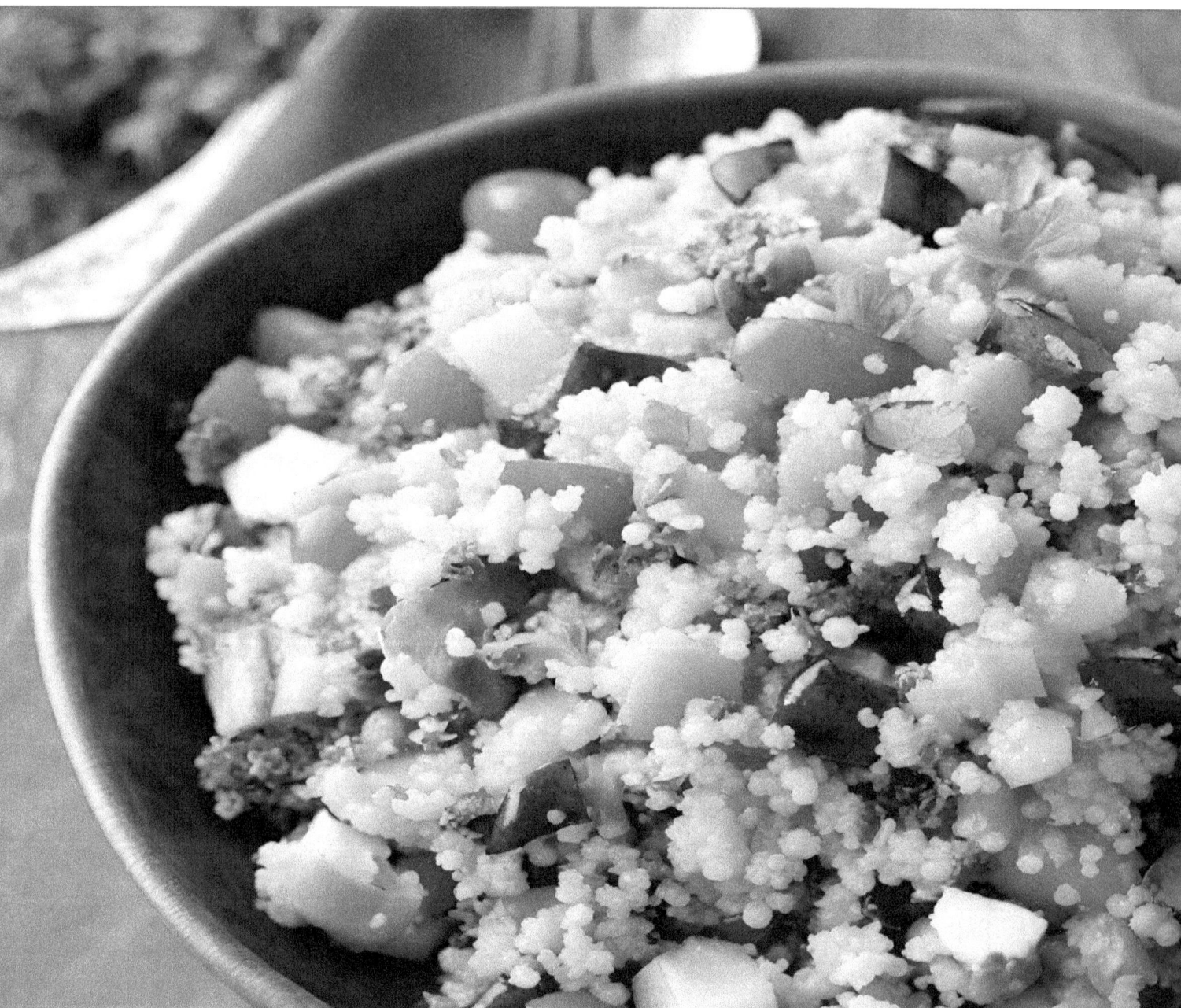

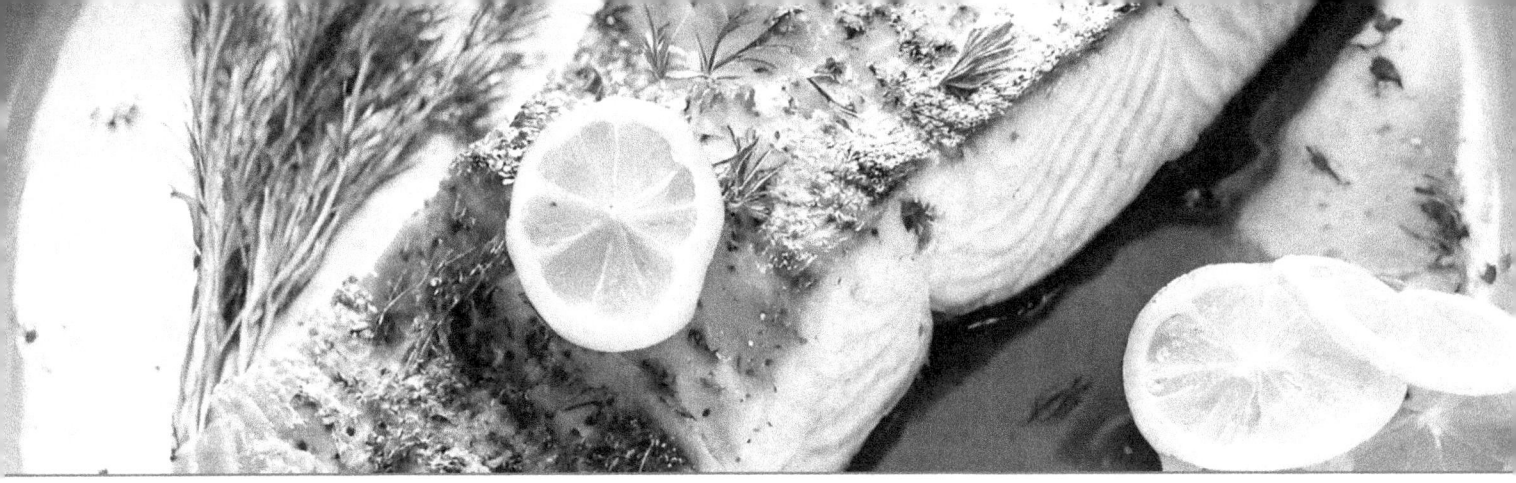

13. Baked Salmon with Dill

Benefits: Salmon is an excellent source of omega-3 fatty acids and high-quality protein.

Servings: 2

Prep/Cook Time: 25 Minutes

Ingredients:

- 2 salmon fillets (4-6 ounces each)
- 1 lemon, sliced
- 2 teaspoons fresh dill, chopped
- Salt and pepper to taste.

Cooking Instructions:

1. Preheat the oven to 350°F (175°C).
2. Place salmon fillets on a baking sheet.
3. Season with salt and pepper, then sprinkle fresh dill on top.
4. Lay lemon slices over the salmon.
5. Bake for about 15-20 minutes, or until the salmon flakes easily with a fork.

Nutritional Information (per serving): Approximately 300 calories, 30g protein, 0g carbohydrates, 0g fiber, 0g sugar, 20g fat, 70mg sodium.

Modification Tip: Use a phosphate binder before the meal to reduce phosphorus absorption. Adjust portion size based on individual dietary restrictions.

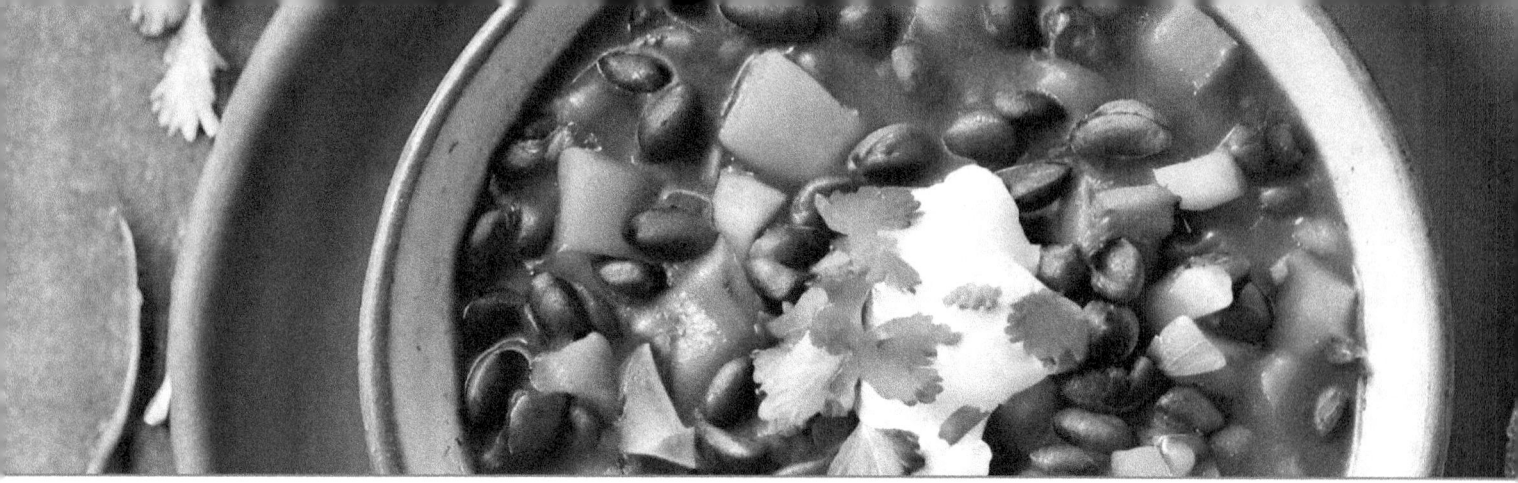

14. Black Bean and Vegetable Soup

Benefits: This soup offers fiber and plant-based protein while keeping phosphorus and potassium in check.

Servings: 4

Ingredients:

- 2 cans (15 ounces each) low-sodium black beans, drained and rinsed
- 1 cup corn kernels (fresh or frozen)
- 1 cup zucchini, diced
- 1 cup carrots, diced
- 1/2 cup red onion, chopped
- 4 cups low-sodium vegetable broth
- 1 teaspoon cumin
- Salt and pepper to taste.

Prep/Cook Time: 30 Minutes

Cooking Instructions:

1. In a large pot, combine black beans, corn, zucchini, carrots, red onion, and vegetable broth.
2. Bring to a boil, then reduce heat to simmer.
3. Add cumin, salt, and pepper. Cook for about 20 minutes, or until vegetables are tender.

Nutritional Information (per serving): Approximately 230 calories, 10g protein, 47g carbohydrates, 11g fiber, 7g sugar, 1g fat, 220mg sodium.

Modification Tip: If potassium is a concern, choose lower-potassium vegetables such as green beans or cauliflower. Also, consider using a phosphate binder before the meal.

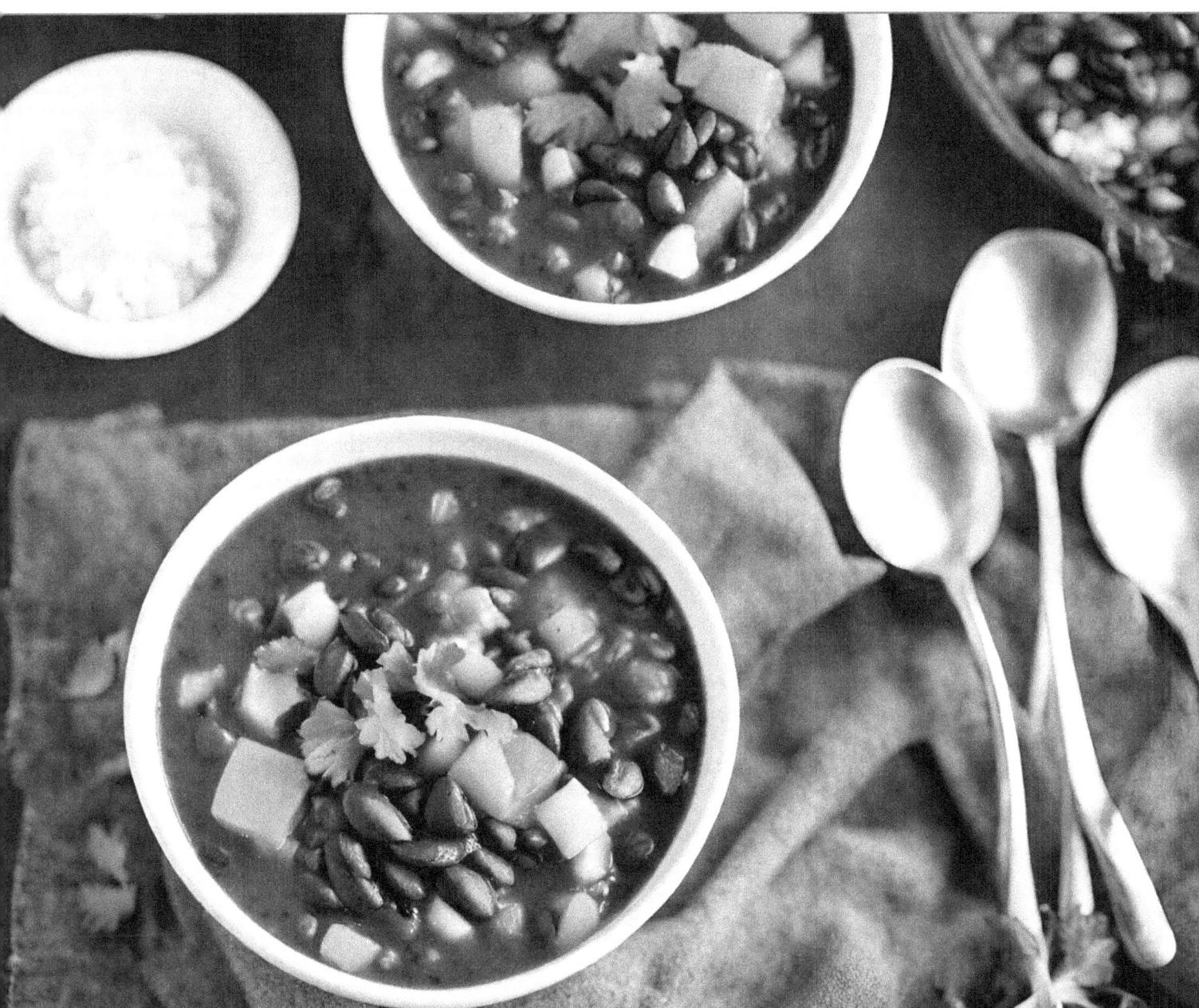

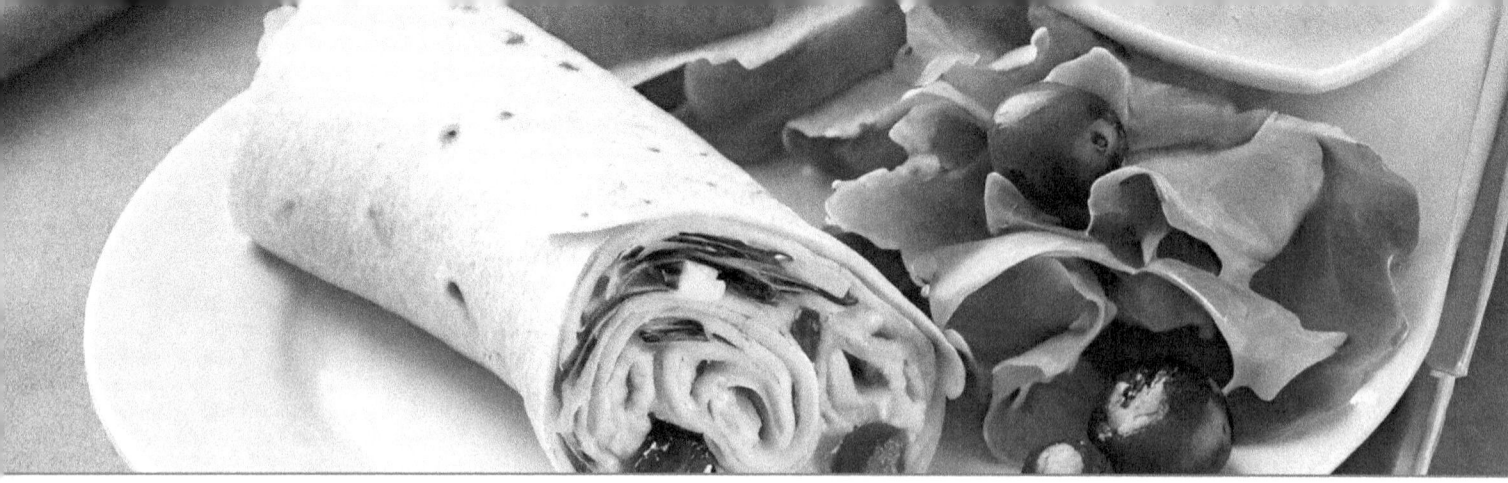

15. Turkey and Cranberry Wrap

Benefits: This wrap offers lean protein with a hint of cranberry sweetness.

Servings: 2   **Prep/Cook Time: 15 Minutes**

Ingredients:

- 8 ounces turkey breast, sliced
- 4 whole-grain tortillas
- 1/4 cup low-sodium cranberry sauce
- 1 cup fresh spinach leaves

Cooking Instructions:

1. Lay out tortillas and spread 1 tablespoon of cranberry sauce on each.
2. Divide turkey slices evenly among the tortillas.
3. Add fresh spinach leaves.
4. Roll up the tortillas, and they're ready to serve.

Nutritional Information (per serving): Approximately 300 calories, 20g protein, 45g carbohydrates, 6g fiber, 10g sugar, 4g fat, 300mg sodium.

Modification Tip: For lower sodium, choose low-sodium turkey and cranberry sauce. If potassium is a concern, consider using a small amount of cranberry sauce or choose a phosphate binder.

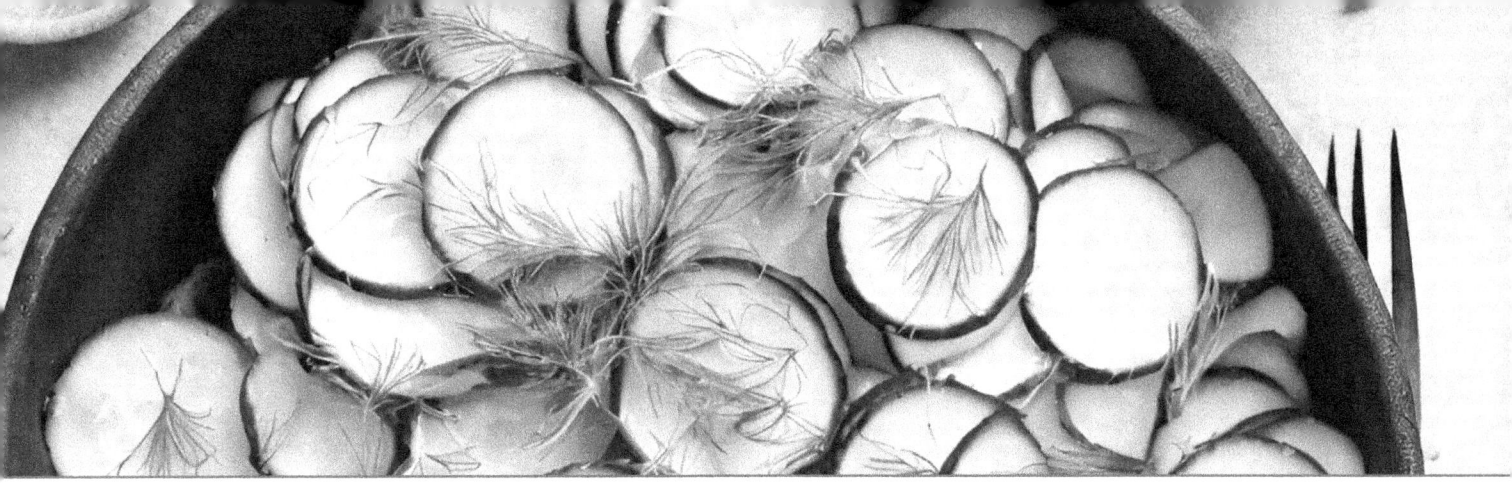

16. Cucumber and Dill Salad

Benefits: This refreshing salad is low in phosphorus and potassium, making it a kidney-friendly side dish.

Servings: 4

Prep/Cook Time: 10 Minutes

Ingredients:

- 2 cucumbers, thinly sliced
- 1/4 cup fresh dill, chopped
- 1/4 cup low-fat sour cream
- 2 tablespoons white wine vinegar
- Salt and pepper to taste

Cooking Instructions:

1. In a bowl, combine sliced cucumbers and chopped dill.
2. In a separate bowl, whisk together sour cream, white wine vinegar, salt, and pepper.
3. Pour the dressing over the cucumbers and dill and toss to coat.

Nutritional Information (per serving): Approximately 60 calories, 1g protein, 7g carbohydrates, 2g fiber, 3g sugar, 3g fat, 15mg sodium.

Modification Tip: To further reduce sodium, use low-sodium sour cream. If potassium is a concern, reduce the portion size.

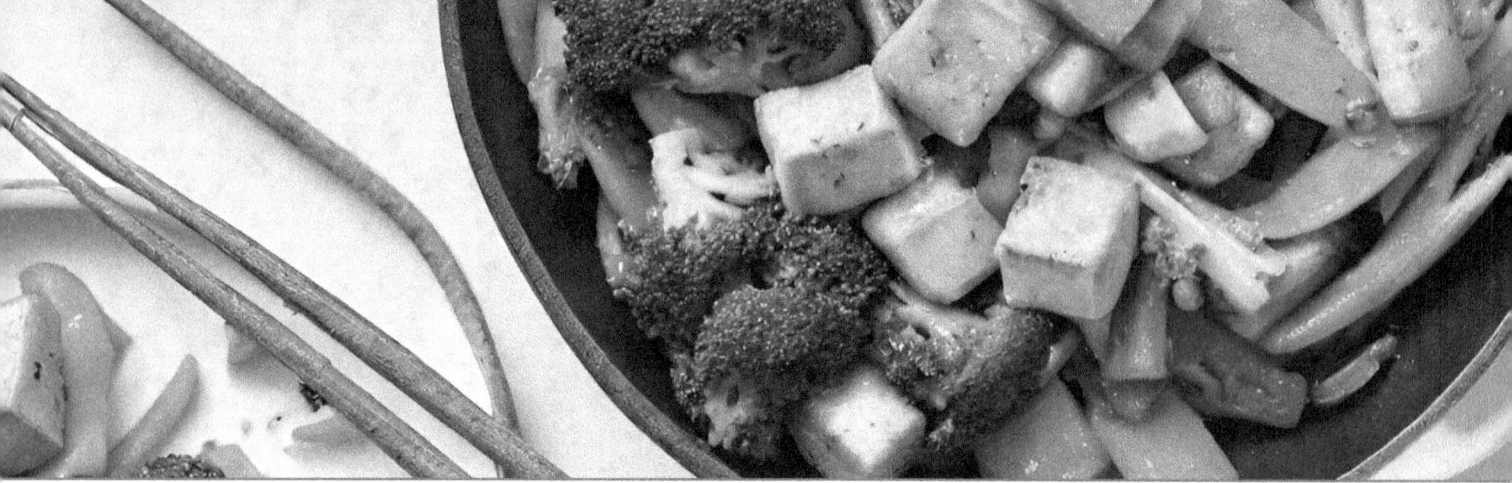

17. Vegetable Stir-Fry with Tofu

Benefits: This stir-fry is rich in plant-based protein, low in phosphorus and potassium, and packed with vegetables.

Servings: 2

Prep/Cook Time: 30 Minutes

Ingredients:

- 1 cup firm tofu, cubed
- 2 cups mixed vegetables (e.g., bell peppers, broccoli, snap peas)
- 2 cloves garlic, minced
- 1 tablespoon low-sodium soy sauce
- 1 tablespoon sesame oil
- 1 teaspoon ginger, minced
- Brown rice (optional, for serving

Cooking Instructions:

1. In a wok or large skillet, heat sesame oil over medium-high heat.
2. Add minced garlic and ginger and sauté for about 1 minute.
3. Add tofu and cook until lightly browned.
4. Add mixed vegetables and continue stir-frying until they are tender.
5. Pour in low-sodium soy sauce and cook for another 2 minutes.
6. Serve on its own or over brown rice.

Nutritional Information (per serving): Approximately 250 calories, 15g protein, 14g carbohydrates, 4g fiber, 5g sugar, 14g fat, 350mg sodium.

Modification Tip: If potassium is a concern, select lower-potassium vegetables like cabbage or green beans. You can also use a phosphate binder before the meal.

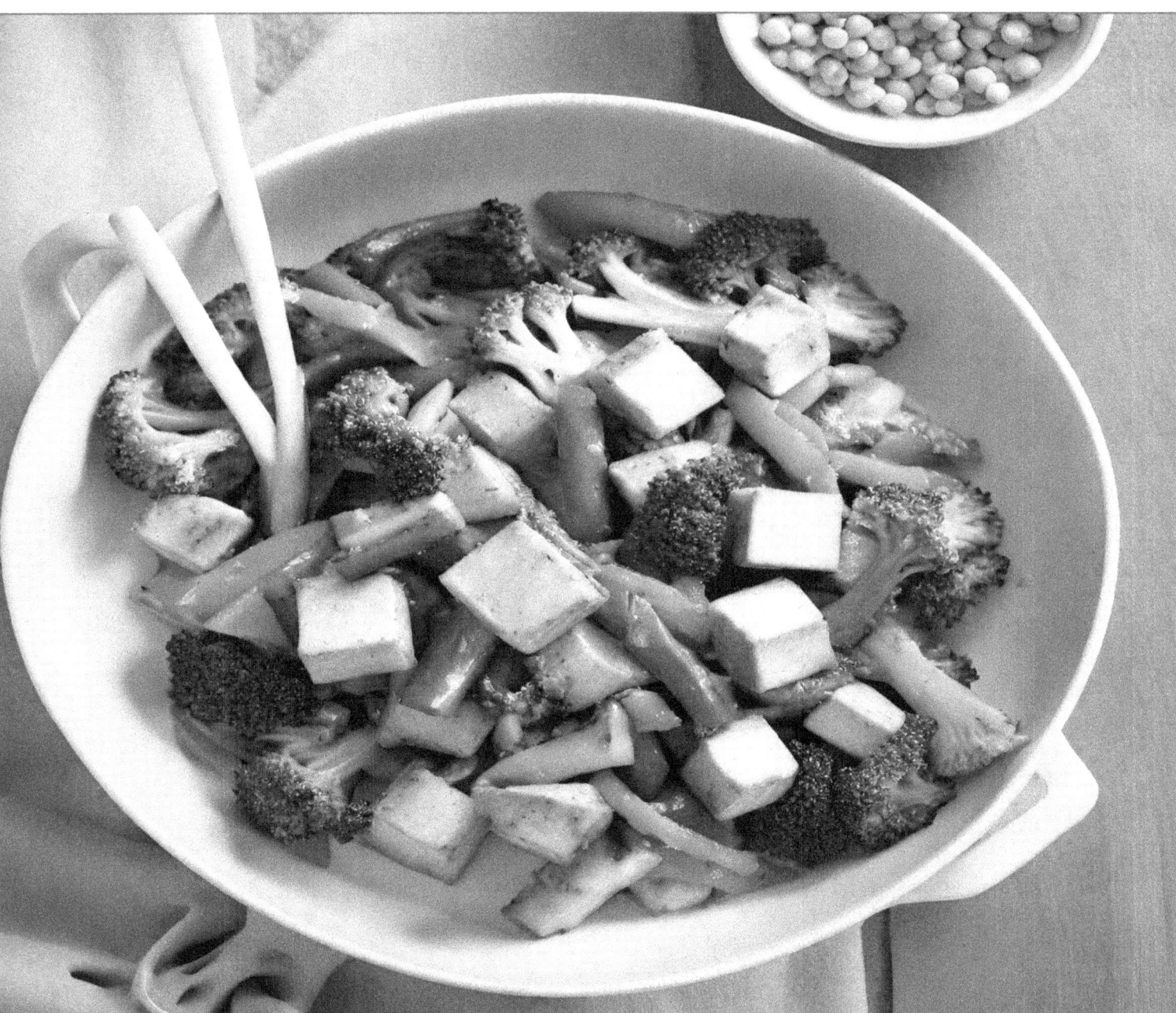

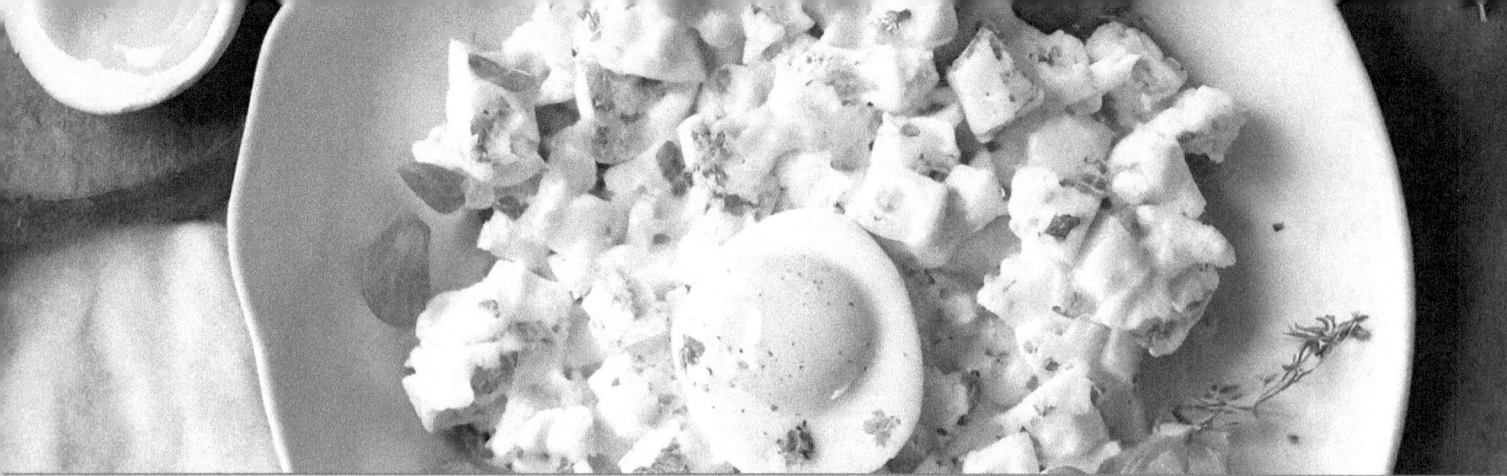

18. Egg Salad with Fresh Herbs

Benefits: This egg salad is a protein-rich, low-phosphorus option that incorporates fresh herbs for added flavor.

Servings: 2

Ingredients:

- 4 hard-boiled eggs, chopped
- 2 tablespoons low-fat mayonnaise
- 1 tablespoon fresh chives, chopped
- 1 tablespoon fresh parsley, chopped
- Salt and pepper to taste

Prep/Cook Time: 20 Minutes

Cooking Instructions:

1. In a bowl, combine chopped hard-boiled eggs, low-fat mayonnaise, fresh chives, and fresh parsley.
2. Mix well and season with salt and pepper to taste.

Nutritional Information (per serving): Approximately 180 calories, 14g protein, 3g carbohydrates, 0g fiber, 2g sugar, 12g fat, 190mg sodium.

Modification Tip: Use low-sodium mayonnaise and reduce the portion size if you need to limit sodium. Consider using a phosphate binder before the meal to reduce phosphorus absorption.

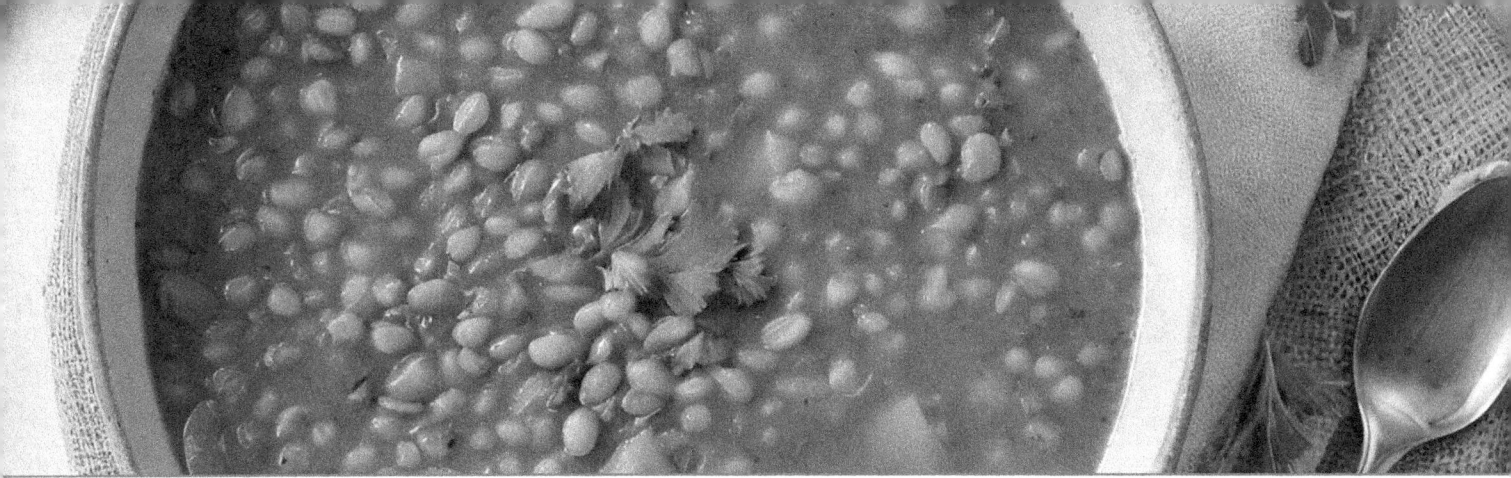

19. Lentil Soup

Benefits: Lentil soup provides plant-based protein and is typically low in phosphorus and potassium.

Servings: 4

Prep/Cook Time: 40 Minutes

Ingredients:

- 1 cup dried green or brown lentils
- 6 cups low-sodium vegetable broth
- 1 cup carrots, diced
- 1 cup celery, diced
- 1 cup onion, chopped
- 2 cloves garlic, minced
- 1 teaspoon cumin
- Salt and pepper to taste

Cooking Instructions:

1. Rinse lentils and pick out any debris.
2. In a large pot, combine lentils, vegetable broth, carrots, celery, onion, and minced garlic.
3. Bring to a boil, then reduce heat and simmer for about 30-40 minutes, or until lentils and vegetables are tender.
4. Season with cumin, salt, and pepper to taste.

Nutritional Information (per serving): Approximately 250 calories, 15g protein, 42g carbohydrates, 10g fiber, 6g sugar, 1g fat, 60mg sodium.

Modification Tip: Ensure you choose low-sodium vegetable broth and consider using a phosphate binder before the meal.

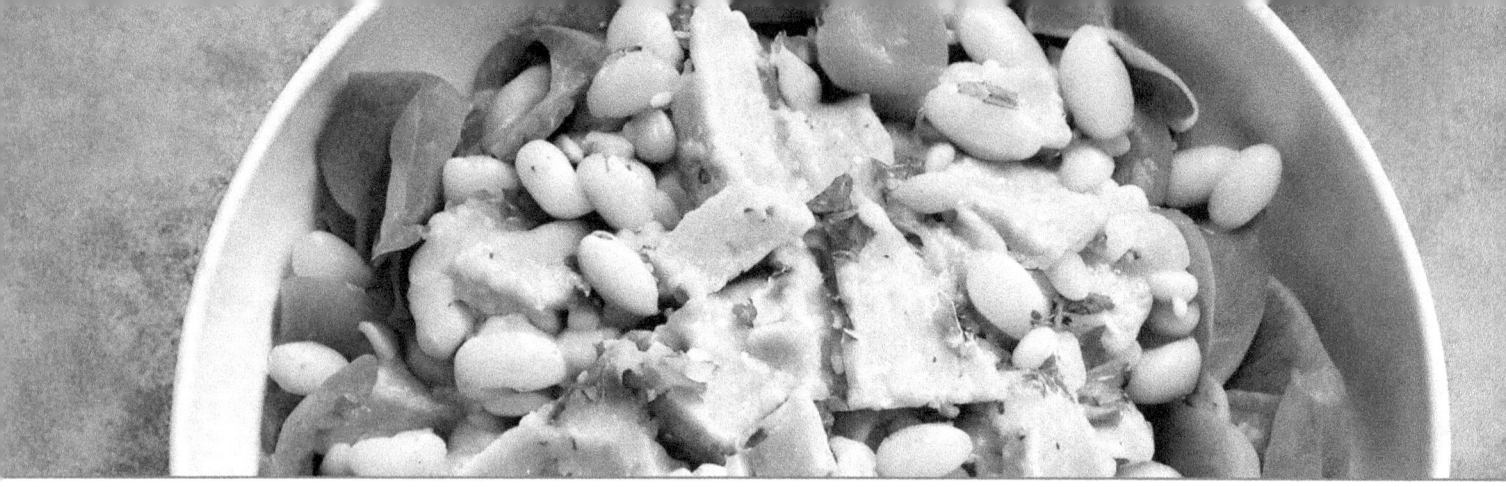

20. Tuna and White Bean Salad

Benefits: This salad combines the protein of tuna with the fiber and nutrients of white beans.

Servings: 2

Prep/Cook Time: 15 Minutes

Ingredients:

- 1 can (5 ounces) low-sodium tuna, drained
- 1 can (15 ounces) low-sodium white beans, drained and rinsed
- 1/2 cup red bell pepper, diced
- 1/4 cup red onion, finely chopped
- 1/4 cup fresh parsley, chopped
- 2 tablespoons olive oil
- 2 tablespoons lemon juice

Cooking Instructions:

1. In a large bowl, combine drained tuna, white beans, diced red bell pepper, chopped red onion, and fresh parsley.
2. In a separate bowl, whisk together olive oil, lemon juice, salt, and pepper.
3. Pour the dressing over the salad and toss to combine.

Ingredients:

- Salt and pepper to taste

Nutritional Information (per serving): Approximately 320 calories, 25g protein, 30g carbohydrates, 9g fiber, 3g sugar, 12g fat, 20mg sodium.

Modification Tip: Ensure you use low-sodium tuna and white beans. To reduce sodium further, consider using a phosphate binder before the meal. If potassium is a concern, reduce the portion size and opt for lower-potassium vegetables like green beans.

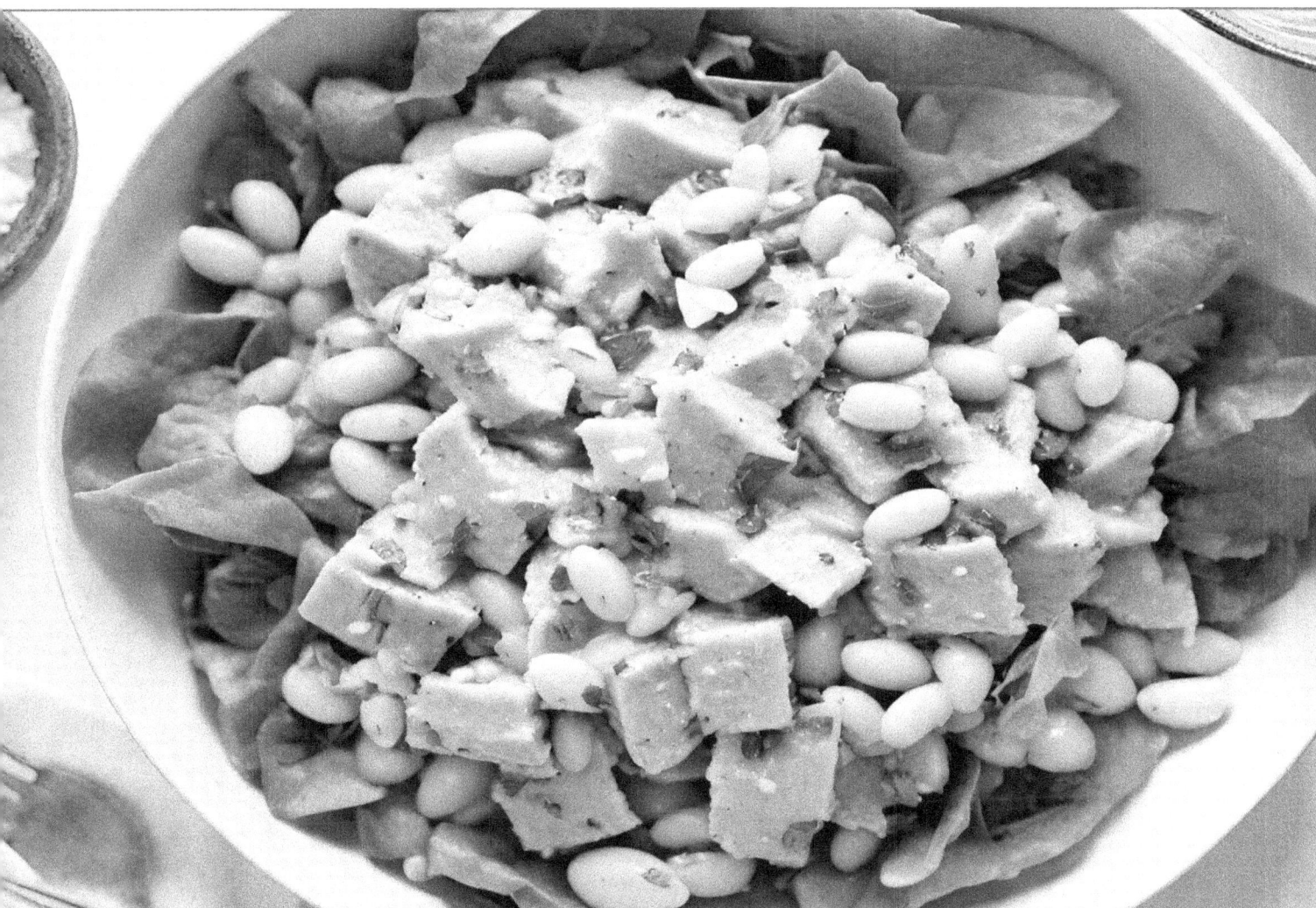

1.3 Dinner Recipes

21. Grilled Lemon Herb Shrimp

22. Baked Cod with Roasted Vegetables

23. Lemon and Herb Roasted Chicken

24. Vegetable and Lentil Stir-Fry

25. Stuffed Bell Peppers with Ground Turkey

26. Herbed Quinoa with Roasted Vegetables

27. Sweet Potato and Chickpea Curry

28. Lemon and Garlic Baked Tilapia

29. Ratatouille

30. Chicken and Asparagus Stir-Fry

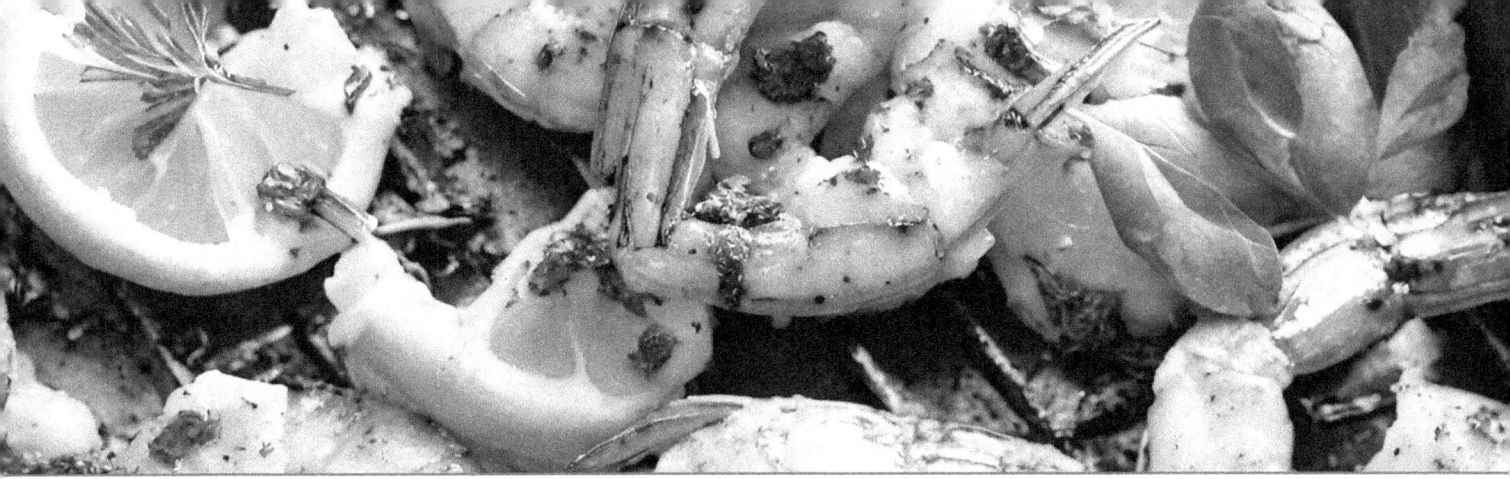

21. Grilled Lemon Herb Shrimp

Benefits: This recipe features lean protein from shrimp, with a zesty lemon herb flavor.

Servings: 2

Prep/Cook Time: 20 Minutes

Ingredients:

- 12 large shrimp (about 6 ounces), peeled and deveined
- 1 lemon (juice and zest)
- 2 cloves garlic, minced
- 1 tablespoon fresh herbs (e.g., basil, parsley), chopped
- Salt and pepper to taste
- Olive oil (for grilling)

Cooking Instructions:

1. In a bowl, combine the lemon juice, lemon zest, minced garlic, fresh herbs, salt, and pepper.
2. Marinate the shrimp in this mixture for 10 minutes.
3. Preheat the grill to medium heat and lightly brush it with olive oil.
4. Grill the shrimp for about 2-3 minutes per side until they are opaque and slightly charred.

Nutritional Information (per serving): Approximately 150 calories, 18g protein, 3g carbohydrates, 1g fiber, 1g sugar, 7g fat, 160mg sodium.

Modification Tip: To reduce sodium, use a salt substitute or less salt in the marinade. For lower phosphorus, consider using a phosphate binder before the meal.

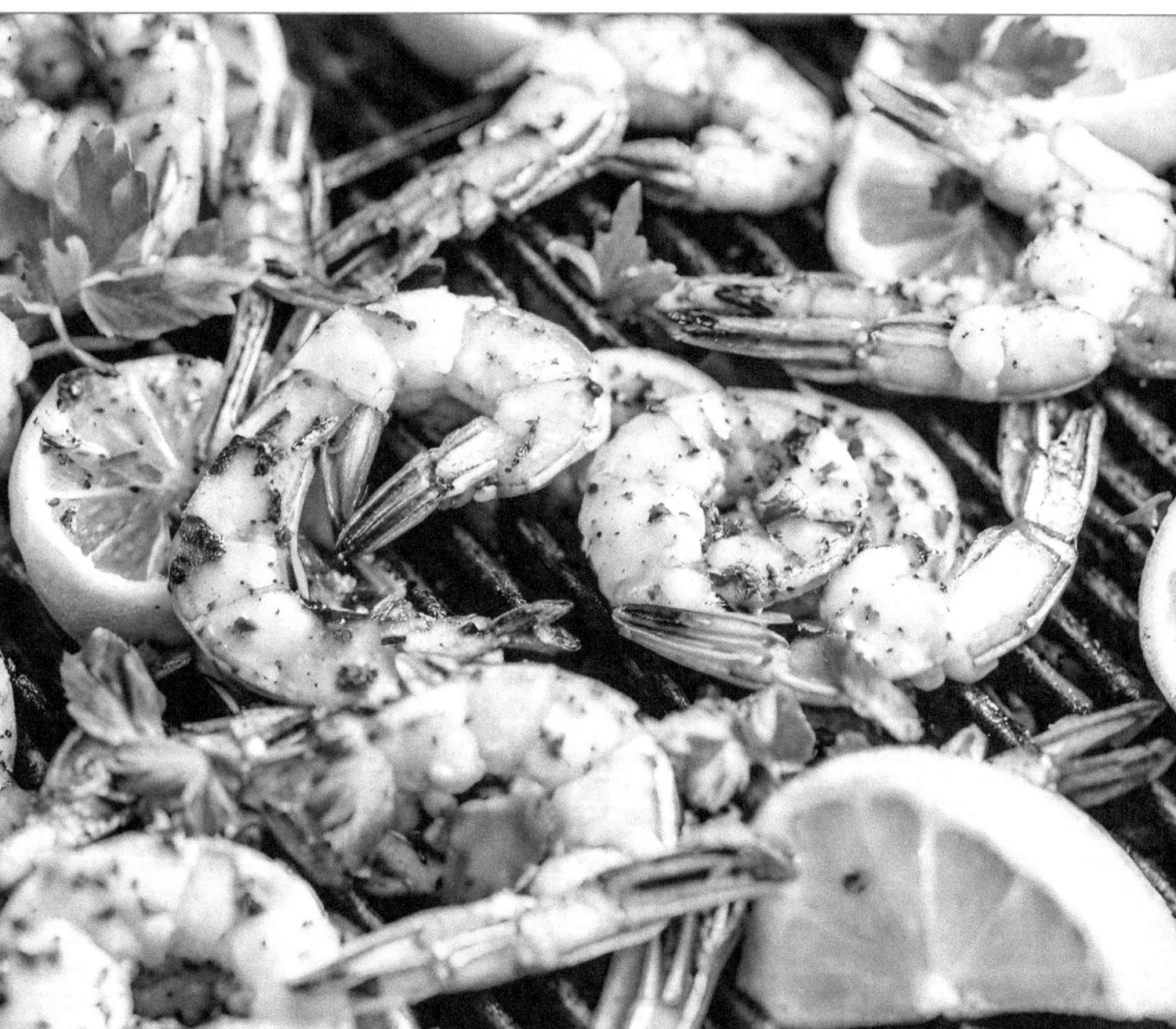

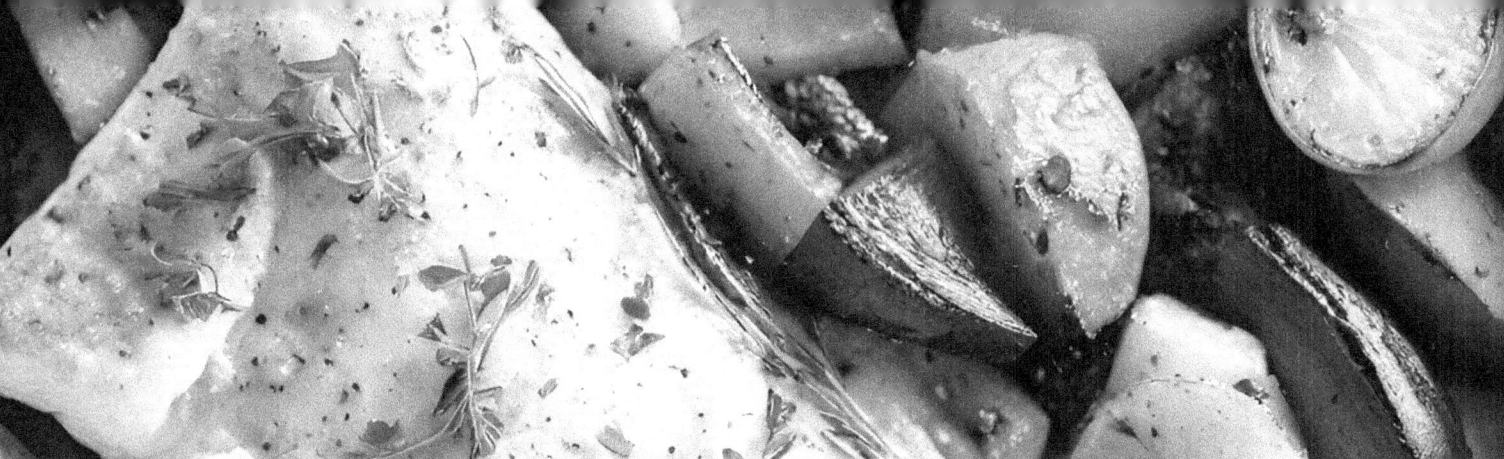

22. Baked Cod with Roasted Vegetables

Benefits: Cod is a mild-flavored, low-phosphorus fish, and this dish is accompanied by fiber-rich roasted vegetables.

Servings: 2

Ingredients:

- 2 cod fillets (about 6 ounces each)
- 2 cups mixed vegetables (e.g., zucchini, bell peppers, carrots), chopped
- 1 tablespoon olive oil
- 1/2 teaspoon dried thyme
- Salt and pepper to taste.

Prep/Cook Time: 30 Minutes

Cooking Instructions:

1. Preheat the oven to 375°F (190°C).
2. Toss the mixed vegetables with olive oil, dried thyme, salt, and pepper.
3. Place the cod fillets on a baking sheet and surround them with the vegetables.
4. Bake for about 20-25 minutes, or until the fish is flaky and the vegetables are tender.

Nutritional Information (per serving): Approximately 220 calories, 30g protein, 10g carbohydrates, 4g fiber, 3g sugar, 7g fat, 70mg sodium.

Modification Tip: For lower sodium, use less salt when seasoning the vegetables and consider using a phosphate binder before the meal.

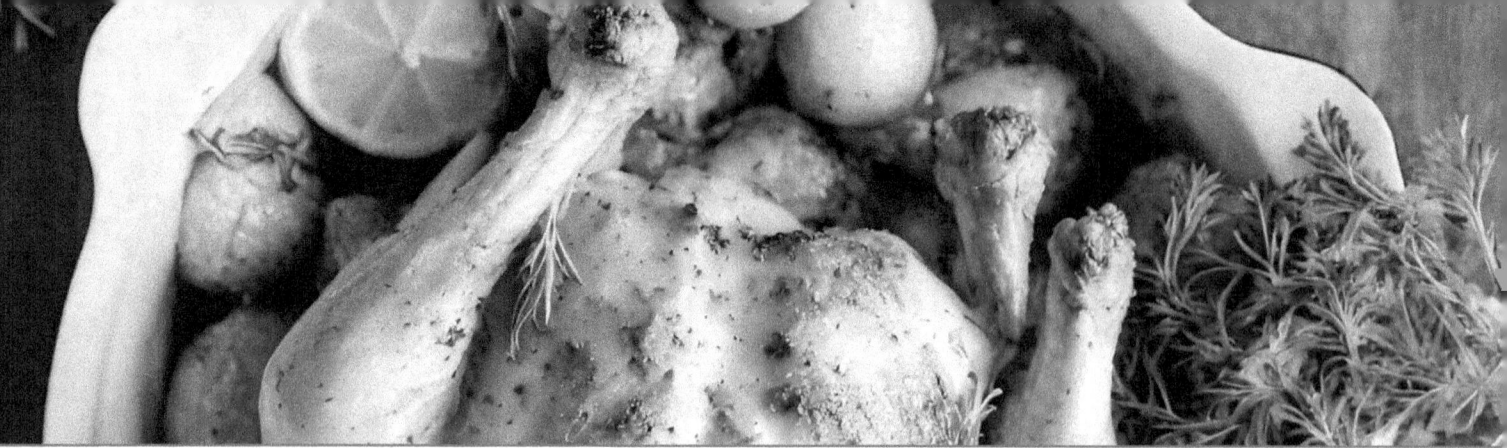

23. Lemon and Herb Roasted Chicken

Benefits: This roasted chicken recipe is flavorful and provides lean protein.

Servings: 2

Ingredients:

- 2 bone-in, skinless chicken thighs (about 6 ounces each)
- 1 lemon (juice and zest)
- 2 cloves garlic, minced
- 1 tablespoon fresh herbs (e.g., rosemary, thyme), chopped
- Salt and pepper to taste
- Olive oil (for roasting)

Prep/Cook Time: 1 Hour

Cooking Instructions:

1. In a bowl, combine the lemon juice, lemon zest, minced garlic, fresh herbs, salt, and pepper.
2. Marinate the chicken thighs in this mixture for 30 minutes.
3. Preheat the oven to 375°F (190°C).
4. Place the marinated chicken thighs in a baking dish, drizzle with olive oil, and roast for about 45-50 minutes, or until they are cooked through and golden brown.

Nutritional Information (per serving): Approximately 230 calories, 25g protein, 3g carbohydrates, 0g fiber, 1g sugar, 13g fat, 180mg sodium.

Modification Tip: For lower sodium, use a salt substitute or less salt in the marinade. To reduce phosphorus, consider using a phosphate binder before the meal.

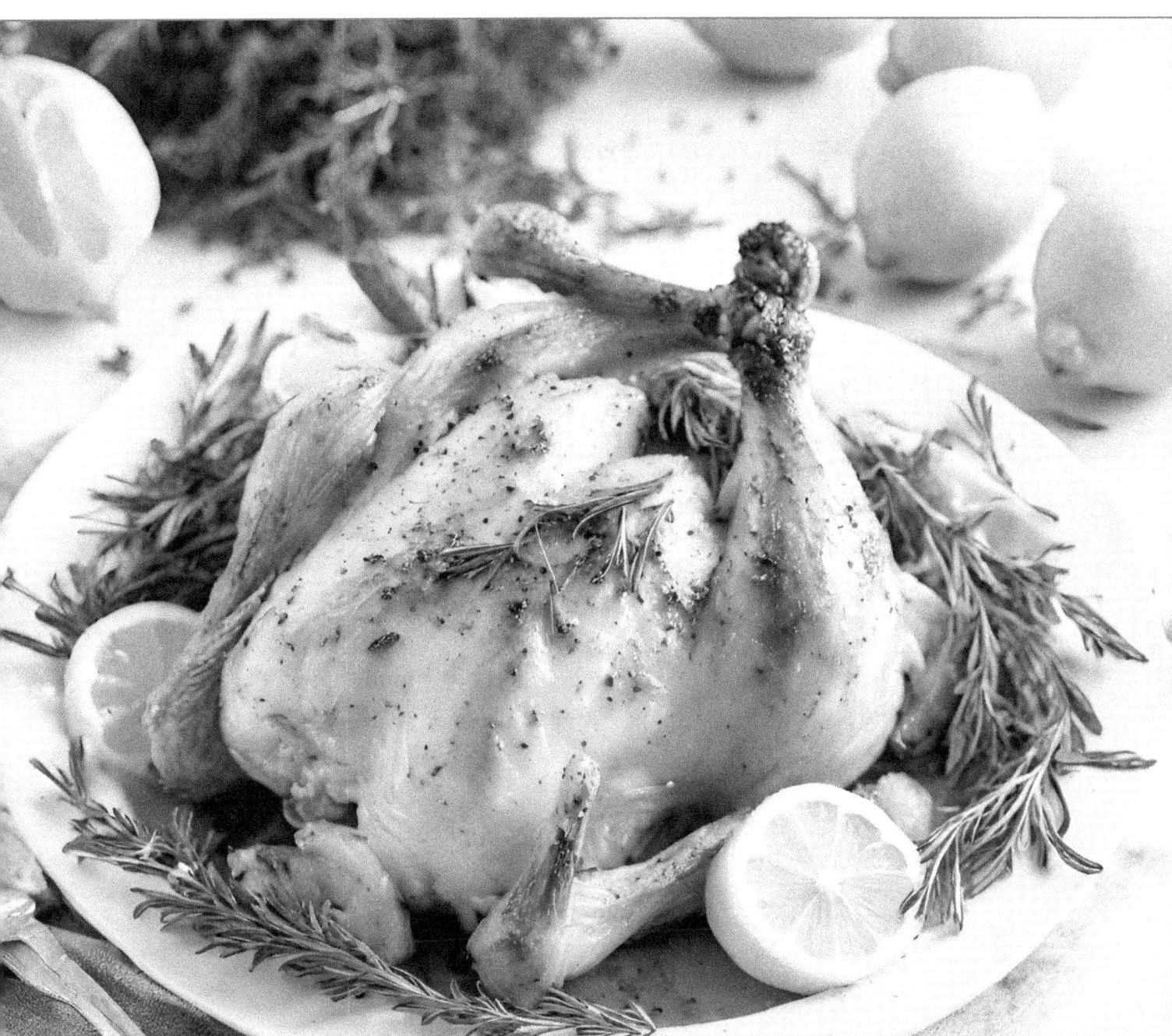

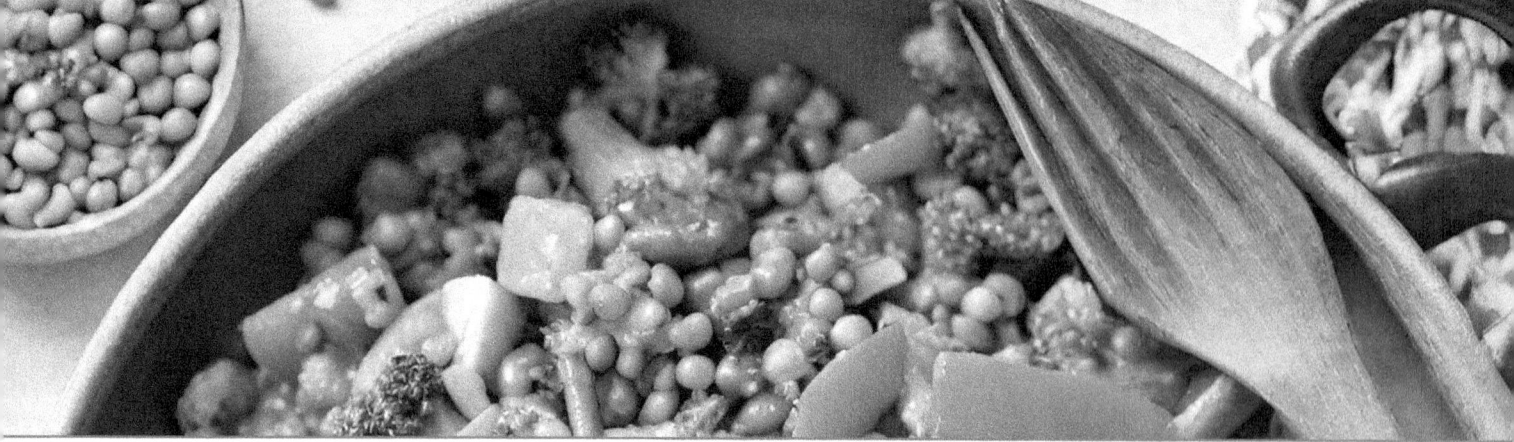

24. Vegetable and Lentil Stir-Fry

Benefits: This stir-fry combines plant-based protein, vegetables, and is low in potassium and phosphorus.

Servings: 2

Ingredients:

- 1 cup dried green or brown lentils
- 2 cups low-sodium vegetable broth
- 2 cups mixed stir-fry vegetables (e.g., bell peppers, broccoli, snap peas)
- 2 cloves garlic, minced
- 1 tablespoon low-sodium soy sauce
- 1 tablespoon sesame oil
- 1 teaspoon ginger, minced

Prep/Cook Time: 30 Minutes

Cooking Instructions:

1. Rinse lentils and pick out any debris.
2. In a saucepan, combine lentils and vegetable broth. Bring to a boil, then reduce heat and simmer for about 20-30 minutes, or until lentils are tender. Drain any excess liquid.
3. In a wok or large skillet, heat sesame oil over medium-high heat.
4. Add minced garlic and ginger, and sauté for about 1 minute.
5. Add mixed vegetables and continue stir-frying until they are tender.
6. Combine cooked lentils with stir-fried vegetables and season with low-sodium soy sauce.
7. Serve on its own or over brown rice.

Ingredients:

- Brown rice (optional, for serving)

Nutritional Information (per serving): Approximately 250 calories, 15g protein, 42g carbohydrates, 10g fiber, 7g sugar, 7g fat, 200mg sodium.

Modification Tip: Ensure you use low-sodium vegetable broth and soy sauce. To reduce phosphorus, consider using a phosphate binder before the meal.

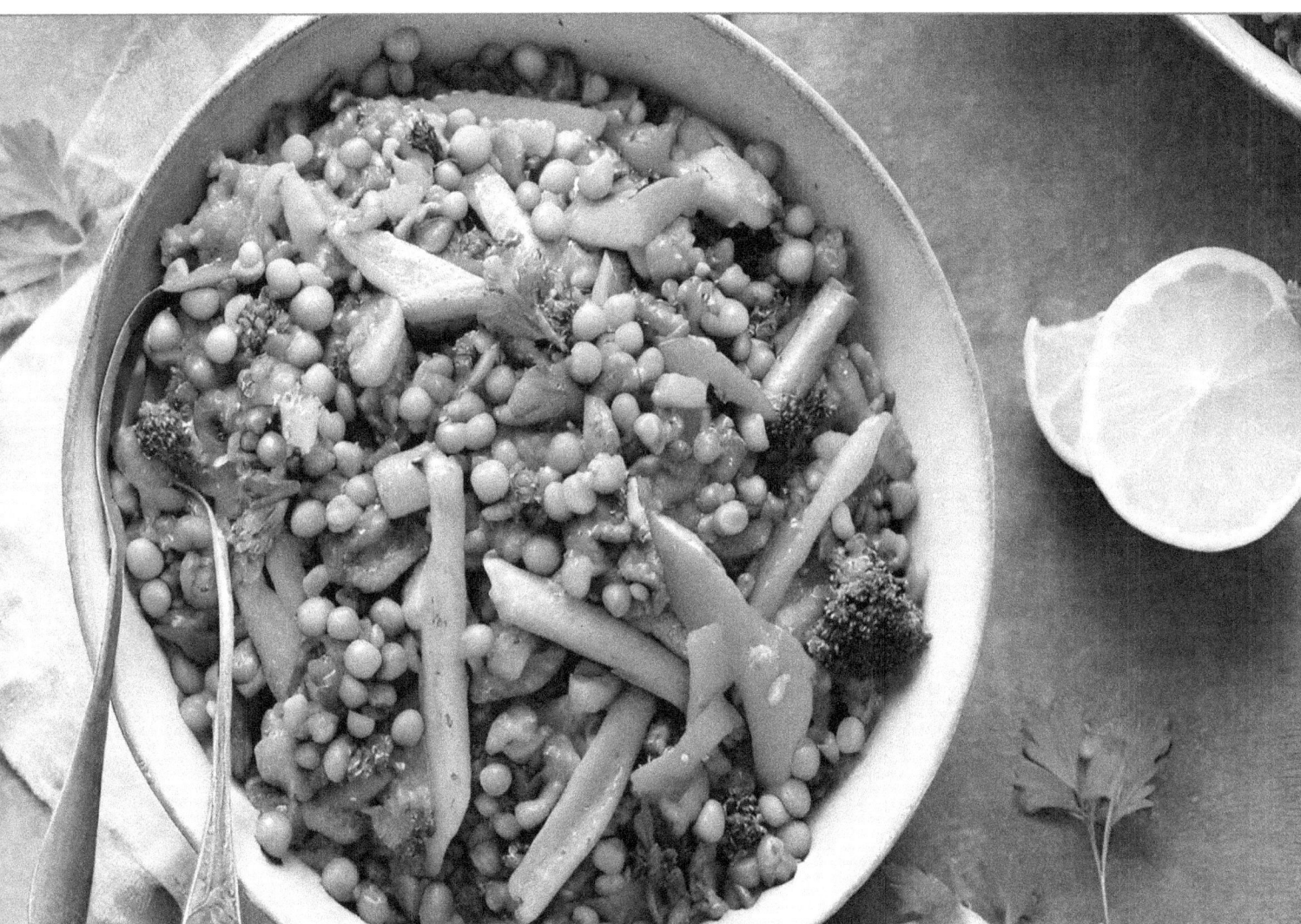

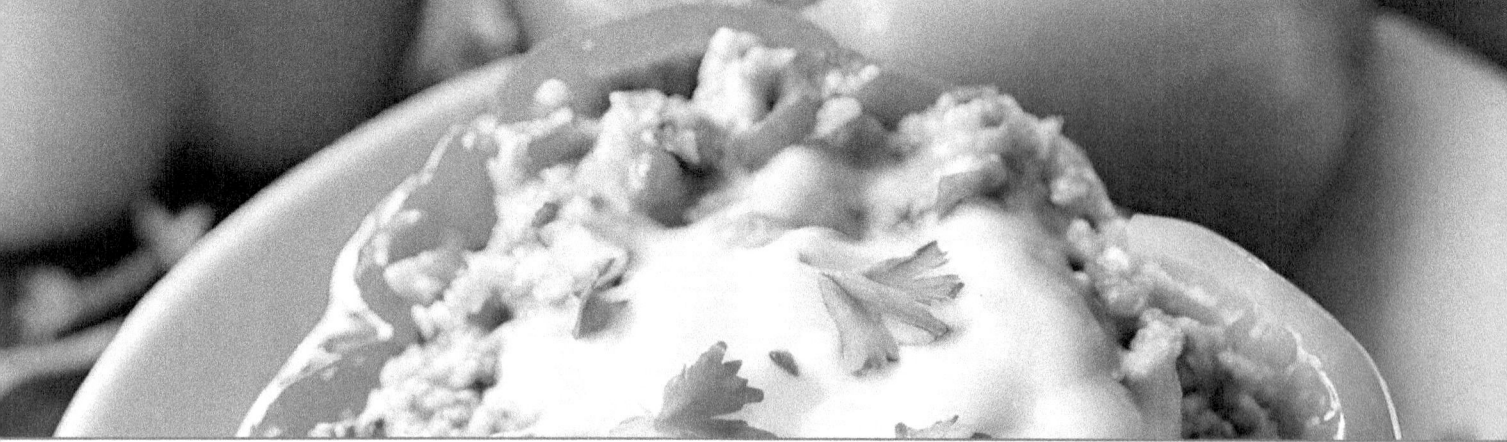

25. Stuffed Bell Peppers with Ground Turkey

Benefits: This dish features lean ground turkey and is low in phosphorus and potassium.

Servings: 2

Ingredients:

- 2 large bell peppers
- 1/2 pound ground turkey
- 1/2 cup brown rice, cooked
- 1/4 cup onion, finely chopped
- 1/4 cup low-sodium tomato sauce
- 1/4 teaspoon garlic powder
- Salt and pepper to taste

Prep/Cook Time: 1 Hour

Cooking Instructions:

1. Preheat the oven to 375°F (190°C).
2. Cut the tops off the bell peppers and remove the seeds and membranes.
3. In a skillet, brown the ground turkey and onions.
4. Stir in cooked brown rice, low-sodium tomato sauce, garlic powder, salt, and pepper.
5. Stuff the bell peppers with the turkey and rice mixture.
6. Place stuffed bell peppers in a baking dish and cover with foil.
7. Bake for about 40-45 minutes, or until the peppers are tender.

Nutritional Information (per serving): Approximately 320 calories, 20g protein, 35g carbohydrates, 4g fiber, 5g sugar, 11g fat, 85mg sodium.

Modification Tip: For lower sodium, use a salt substitute or less salt in the filling. If potassium is a concern, reduce the portion size of the stuffed

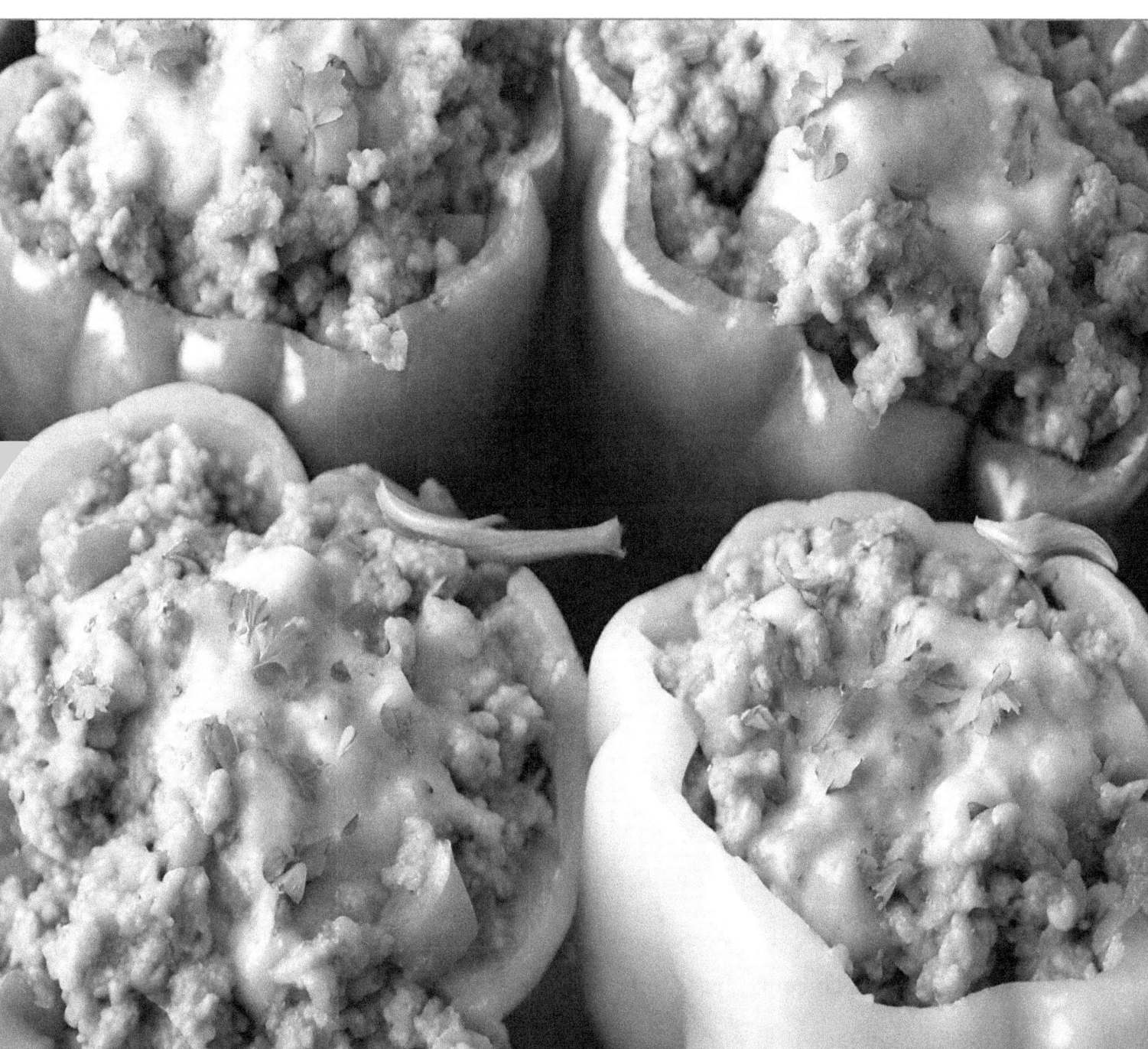

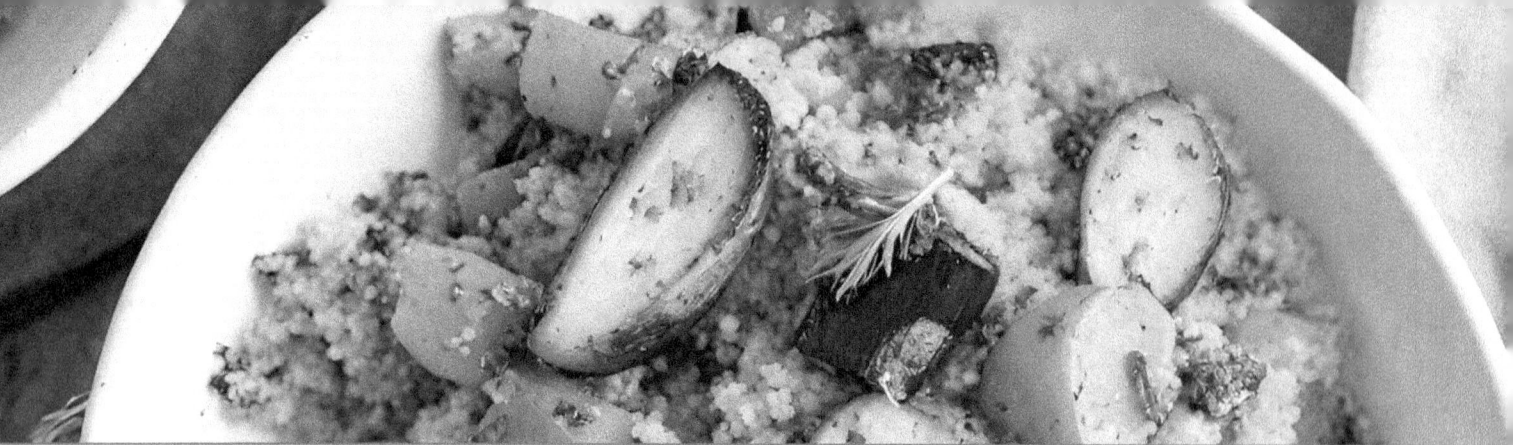

26. Herbed Quinoa with Roasted Vegetables

Benefits: Quinoa offers a complete protein source, and the roasted vegetables provide fiber and vitamins.

Servings: 2

Ingredients:

- 1 cup quinoa, rinsed
- 2 cups water
- 2 cups mixed roasted vegetables (e.g., eggplant, bell peppers, zucchini)
- 1 tablespoon olive oil
- 1 tablespoon fresh herbs (e.g., thyme, oregano), chopped
- Salt and pepper to taste.

Prep/Cook Time: 40 Minutes

Cooking Instructions:

1. Boil 2 cups of water and add quinoa. Simmer for about 15 minutes, or until quinoa is cooked and water is absorbed.
2. Toss mixed roasted vegetables with olive oil, fresh herbs, salt, and pepper.
3. Serve the quinoa with a portion of roasted vegetables on top.

Nutritional Information (per serving): Approximately 260 calories, 7g protein, 45g carbohydrates, 6g fiber, 3g sugar, 7g fat, 20mg sodium.

Modification Tip: Ensure you season the vegetables with less salt to reduce sodium content. If potassium is a concern, choose lower-potassium vegetables like cauliflower or green beans.

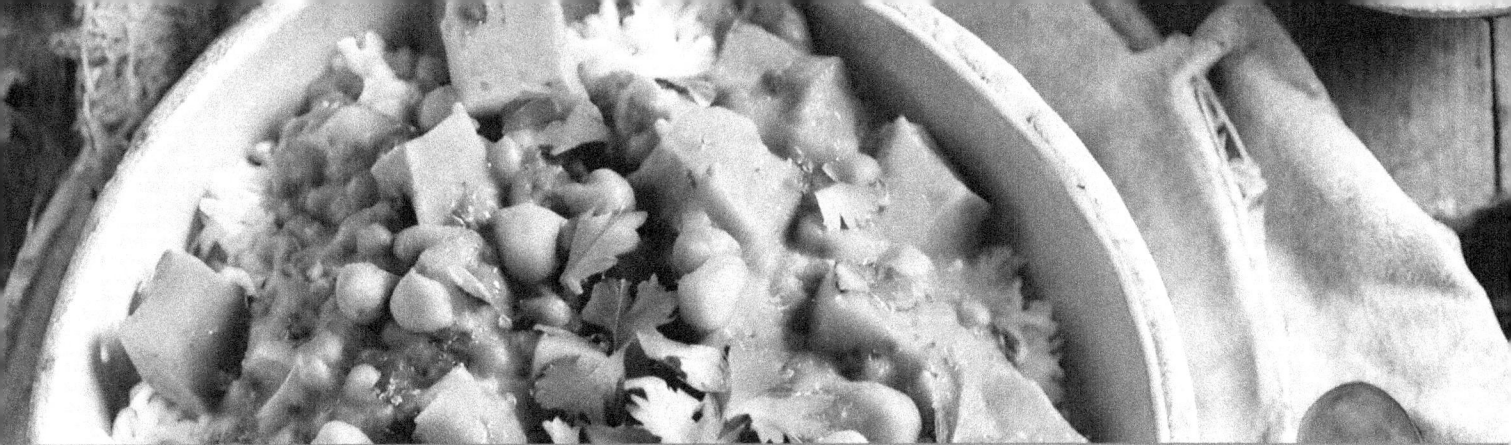

27. Sweet Potato and Chickpea Curry

Benefits: This curry is rich in plant-based protein, fiber, and is a flavorful low-phosphorus and low-potassium option.

Servings: 2

Prep/Cook Time: 40 Minutes

Ingredients:

- 1 large sweet potato, peeled and diced
- 1 can (15 ounces) low-sodium chickpeas, drained and rinsed
- 1/2 cup onion, finely chopped
- 2 cloves garlic, minced
- 1 can (14 ounces) low-sodium diced tomatoes
- 2 tablespoons curry powder
- Salt and pepper to taste.

Cooking Instructions:

1. In a large pot, heat olive oil over medium heat.
2. Add chopped onion and minced garlic, and sauté for about 2 minutes.
3. Stir in diced sweet potato, chickpeas, diced tomatoes, curry powder, salt, and pepper.
4. Add enough water to cover the ingredients, then bring to a boil.
5. Reduce heat and simmer for about 20-25 minutes, or until the sweet potato is tender.

Ingredients:

- 1 tablespoon olive oil

Nutritional Information (per serving): Approximately 280 calories, 11g protein, 51g carbohydrates, 10g fiber, 9g sugar, 5g fat, 180mg sodium.

Modification Tip: To reduce sodium, use a salt substitute or less salt. If potassium is a concern, reduce the portion size.

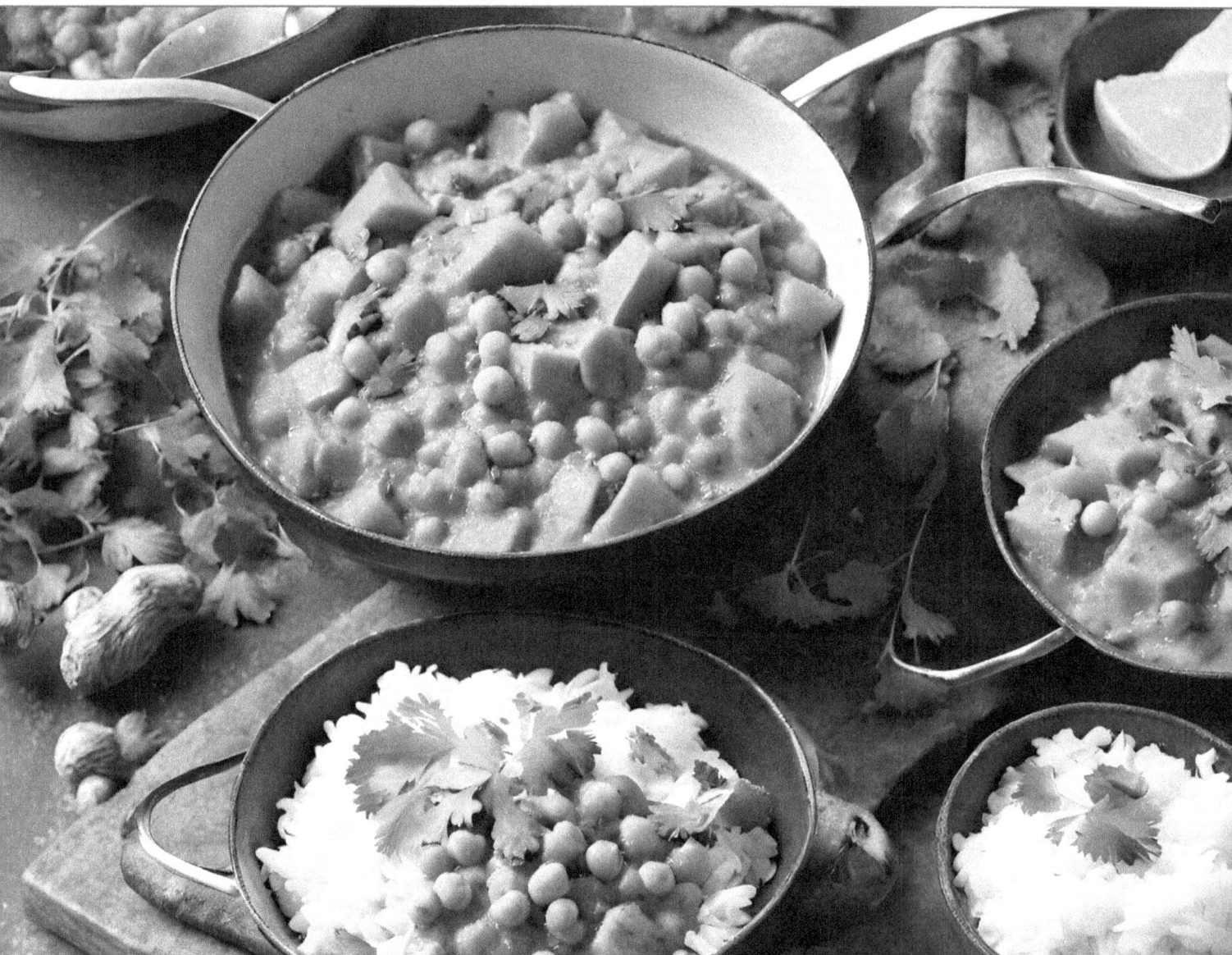

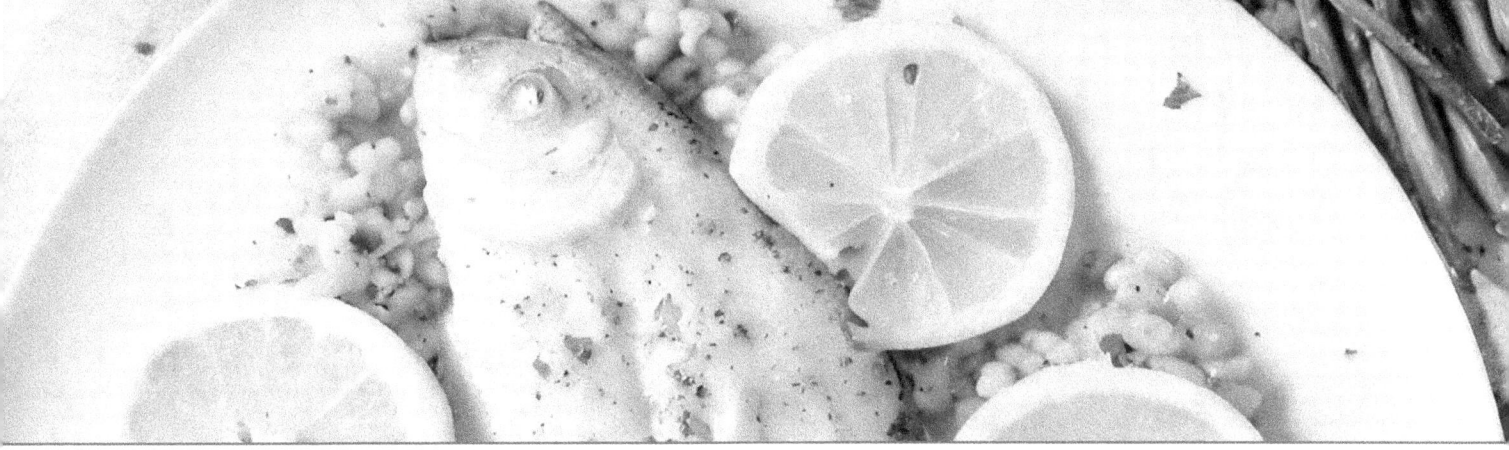

28. Lemon and Garlic Baked Tilapia

Benefits: Tilapia is a mild-flavored, low-phosphorus fish, and this recipe is infused with zesty lemon and garlic.

Servings: 2

Prep/Cook Time: 25 Minutes

Ingredients:

- 2 tilapia fillets (about 6 ounces each)
- 1 lemon (juice and zest)
- 2 cloves garlic, minced
- 1 tablespoon fresh parsley, chopped
- Salt and pepper to taste
- Olive oil (for baking)

Cooking Instructions:

1. Preheat the oven to 375°F (190°C).
2. Place tilapia fillets on a baking sheet.
3. In a bowl, combine the lemon juice, lemon zest, minced garlic, fresh parsley, salt, and pepper.
4. Drizzle the lemon and garlic mixture over the tilapia fillets and drizzle with a touch of olive oil.
5. Bake for about 15-20 minutes, or until the fish flakes easily with a fork.

Nutritional Information (per serving): Approximately 150 calories, 30g protein, 2g carbohydrates, 0g fiber, 1g sugar, 2g fat, 70mg sodium.

Modification Tip: For lower sodium, use a salt substitute or less salt in the lemon and garlic mixture. To reduce phosphorus, consider using a phosphate binder before the meal.

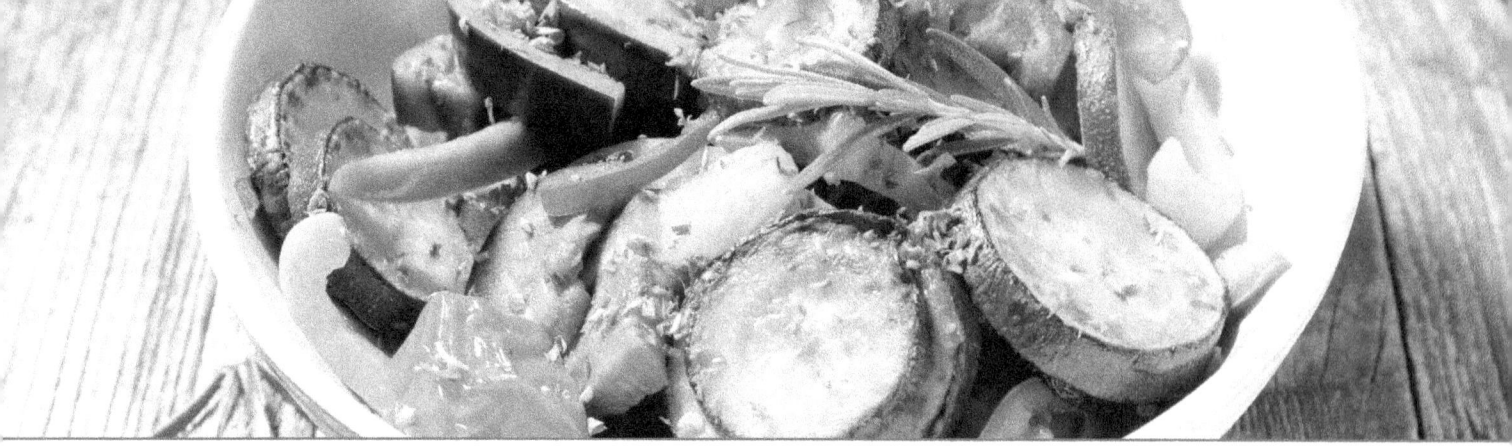

29. Ratatouille

Benefits: Ratatouille is a flavorful vegetable medley that is naturally low in phosphorus and potassium.

Servings: 2

Prep/Cook Time: 45 Minutes

Ingredients:

- 1 small eggplant, diced
- 1 zucchini, diced
- 1 yellow squash, diced
- 1 red bell pepper, diced
- 1 onion, chopped
- 2 cloves garlic, minced
- 1 can (14 ounces) low-sodium diced tomatoes
- 1/2 teaspoon dried thyme
- 1/2 teaspoon dried basil

Cooking Instructions:

1. In a large skillet, heat olive oil over medium heat.
2. Add chopped onion and minced garlic and sauté for about 2 minutes.
3. Stir in diced eggplant, zucchini, yellow squash, red bell pepper, dried thyme, dried basil, salt, and pepper.
4. Cook for about 10-15 minutes, or until the vegetables are tender.
5. Add the can of diced tomatoes and simmer for an additional 10 minutes.

Ingredients:

- 1/2 teaspoon dried basil
- Salt and pepper to taste
- 1 tablespoon olive oil

Nutritional Information (per serving): Approximately 180 calories, 4g protein, 33g carbohydrates, 10g fiber, 13g sugar, 6g fat, 25mg sodium.

Modification Tip: To further reduce sodium, choose low-sodium canned tomatoes and use a salt substitute. If potassium is a concern, consider reducing the portion size.

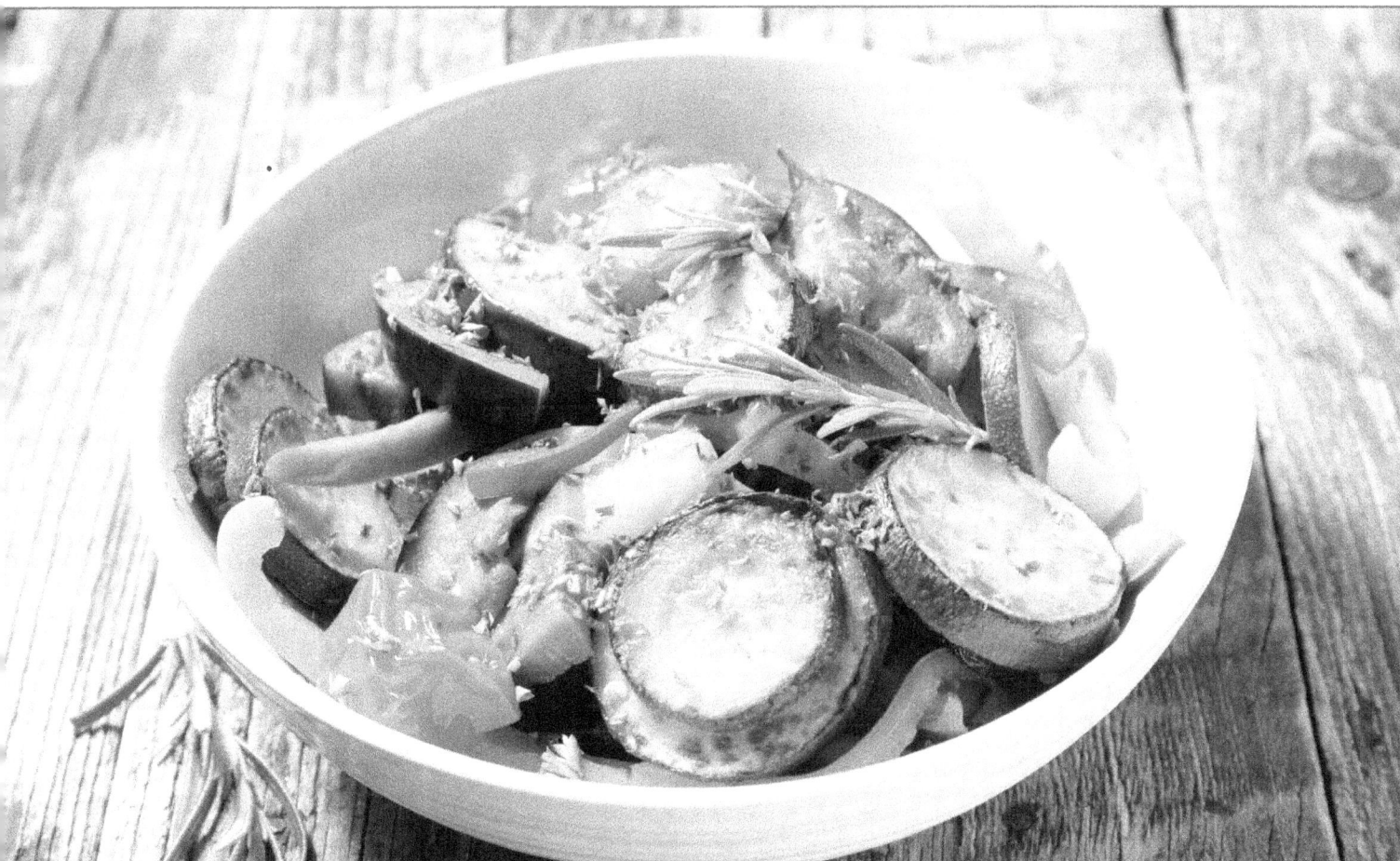

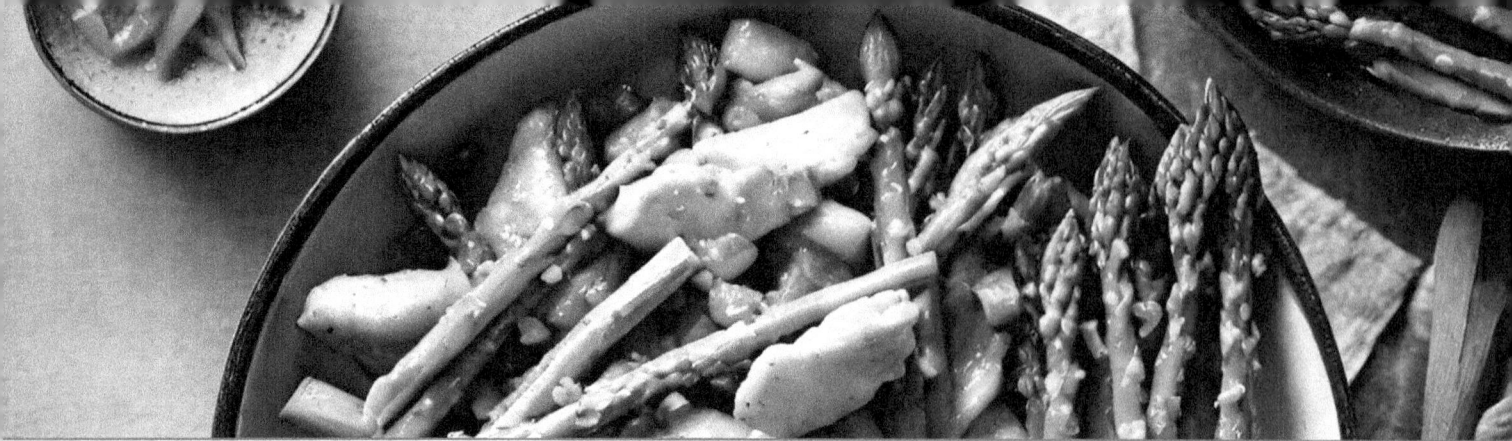

30. Chicken and Asparagus Stir-Fry

Benefits: This stir-fry features lean chicken and asparagus, keeping potassium and phosphorus in check.

Servings: 2

Ingredients:

- 2 boneless, skinless chicken breasts (about 4-6 ounces each), sliced
- 1 bunch asparagus, cut into bite-sized pieces
- 2 cloves garlic, minced
- 2 tablespoons low-sodium soy sauce
- 1 tablespoon olive oil
- Salt and pepper to taste
- 1/4 cup low-sodium chicken broth

Prep/Cook Time: 30 Minutes

Cooking Instructions:

1. In a wok or large skillet, heat olive oil over medium-high heat.
2. Add minced garlic and stir-fry for about 1 minute.
3. Add sliced chicken and cook until it's no longer pink.
4. Add asparagus and continue stir-frying until the asparagus is tender and the chicken is cooked through.
5. Stir in low-sodium soy sauce and low-sodium chicken broth, then simmer for an additional 2 minutes.

Nutritional Information (per serving): Approximately 220 calories, 30g protein, 4g carbohydrates, 2g fiber, 2g sugar, 9g fat, 300mg sodium.

Modification Tip: For lower sodium, use a salt substitute or less low-sodium soy sauce. To reduce phosphorus, consider using a phosphate binder before the meal.

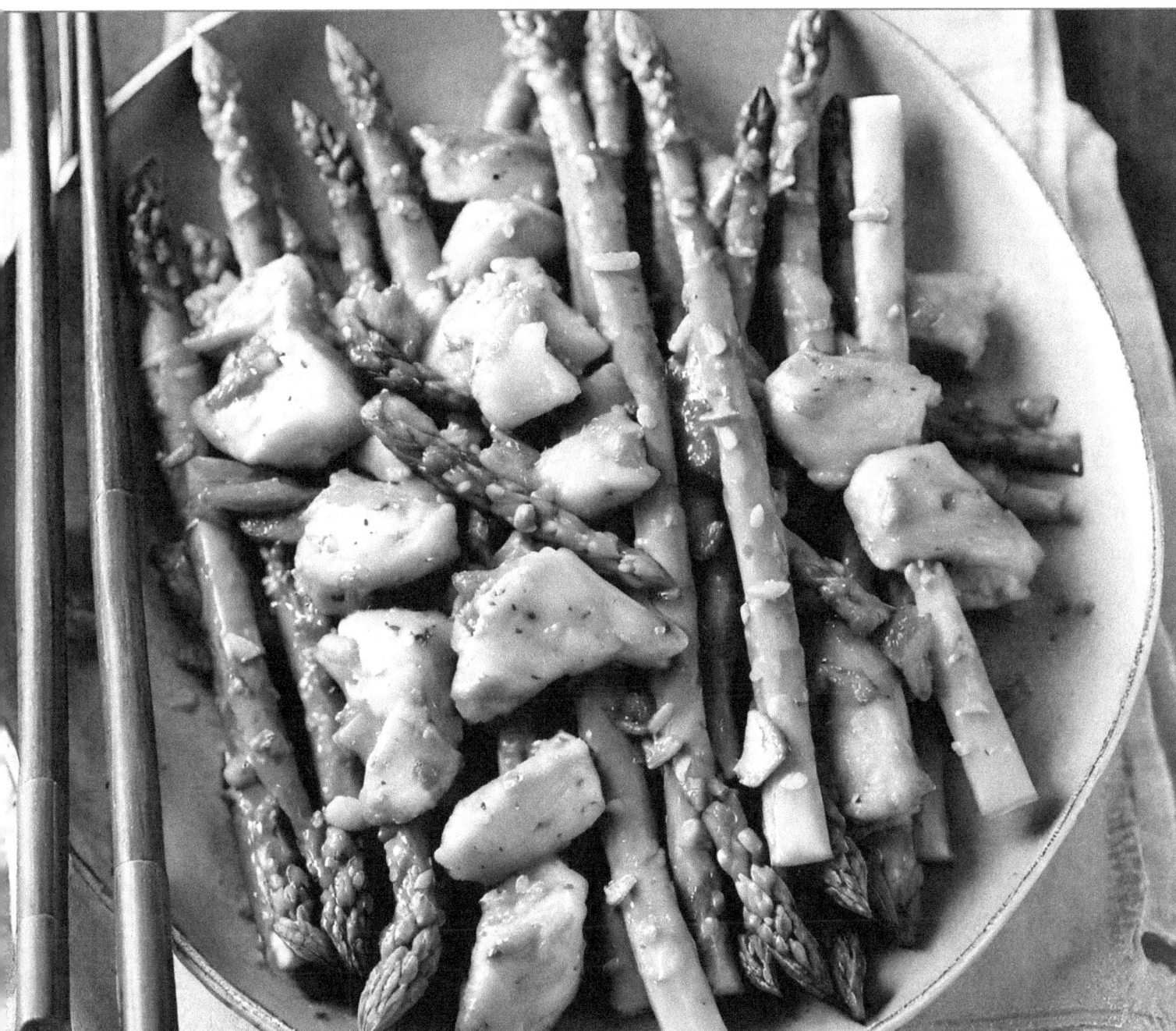

1.4 Snacks

31. Cottage Cheese with Berries

32. Baked Sweet Potato Fries

33. Greek Yogurt Parfait

34. Hummus with Cucumber Slices

35. Rice Cake with Almond Butter

36. Mixed Nuts

37. Celery and Cream Cheese

38. Sliced Apples with Peanut Butter

39. Carrot Sticks with Guacamole

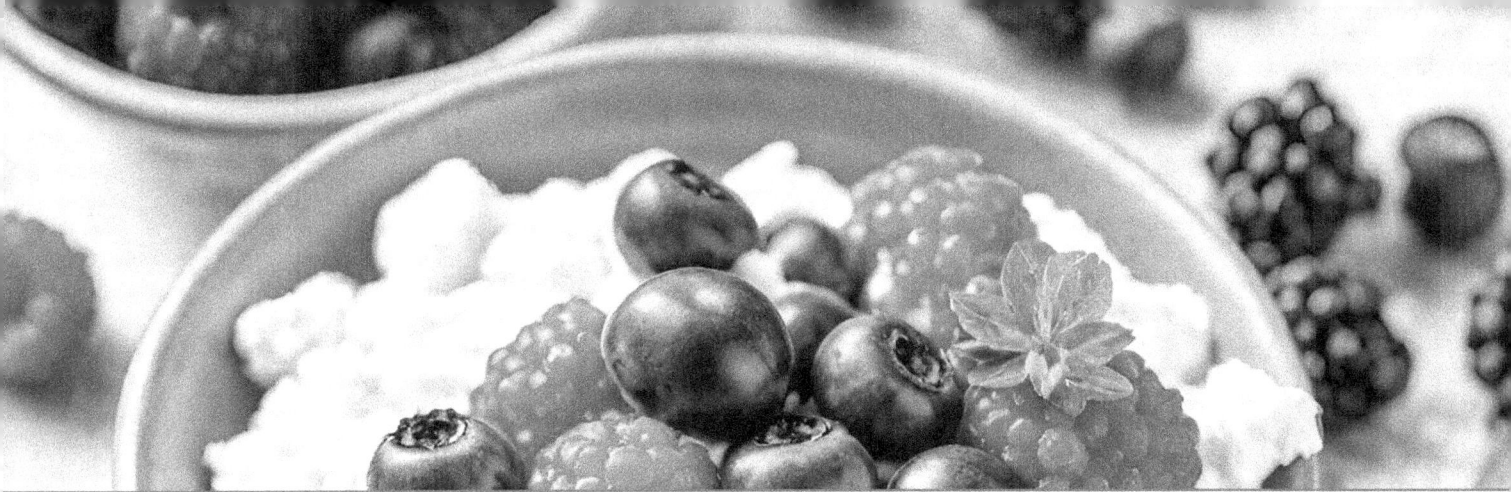

31. Cottage Cheese with Berries

Benefits: This snack is a good source of protein and antioxidants.

Servings: 1

Ingredients:

- 1/2 cup low-fat cottage cheese
- 1/4 cup mixed berries (e.g., blueberries, strawberries)
- 1 teaspoon honey (optional)
- Fresh mint leaves for garnish

Prep/Cook Time: 5 Minutes

Cooking Instructions:

1. In a bowl, place the cottage cheese.
2. Top with mixed berries and drizzle honey if desired.
3. Garnish with fresh mint leaves.

Nutritional Information (per serving): Approximately 150 calories, 15g protein, 10g carbohydrates, 2g fiber, 8g sugar, 4g fat, 300mg sodium.

Modification Tip: For lower sodium, choose a low-sodium cottage cheese. To reduce potassium, decrease the portion of berries or opt for lower-potassium fruits.

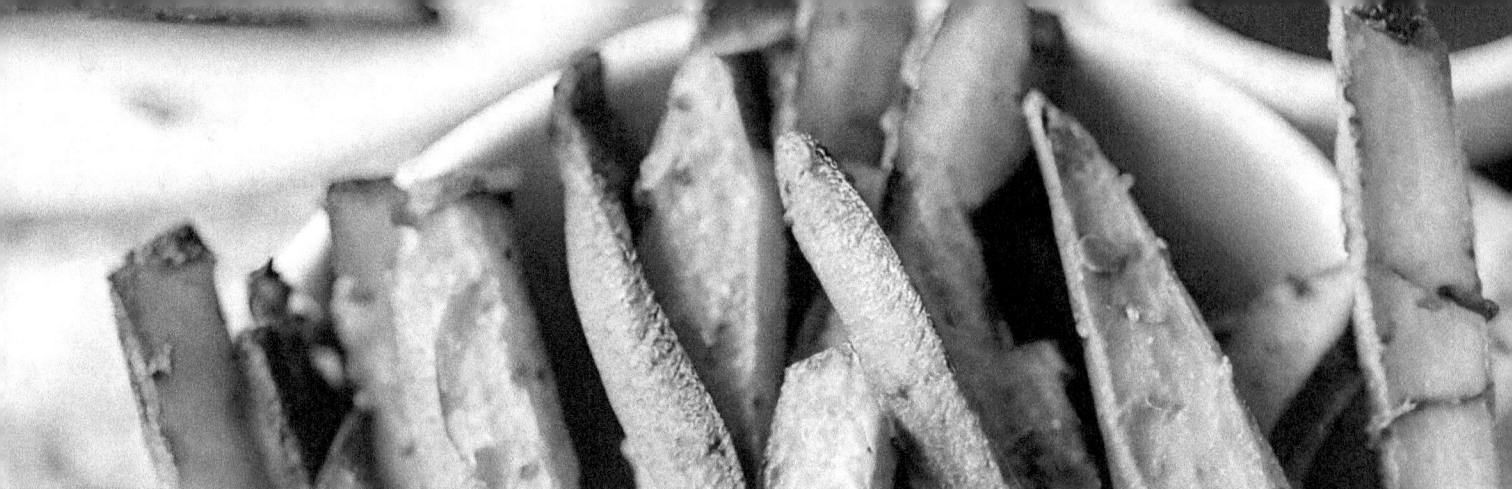

32. Baked Sweet Potato Fries

Benefits: These sweet potato fries are a tasty and low-potassium snack.

Servings: 1

Ingredients:

- 1 medium sweet potato, peeled and cut into fries
- 1 tablespoon olive oil
- 1/2 teaspoon paprika
- Salt and pepper to taste

Prep/Cook Time: 30 Minutes

Cooking Instructions:

1. Preheat the oven to 425°F (220°C).
2. In a bowl, toss sweet potato fries with olive oil, paprika, salt, and pepper.
3. Spread the fries on a baking sheet.
4. Bake for about 20-25 minutes, turning them once, until they are crispy.

Nutritional Information (per serving): Approximately 120 calories, 1g protein, 17g carbohydrates, 3g fiber, 4g sugar, 5g fat, 80mg sodium.

Modification Tip: To reduce sodium, omit the salt or use a salt substitute. To further reduce potassium, consume a smaller portion of sweet potato fries.

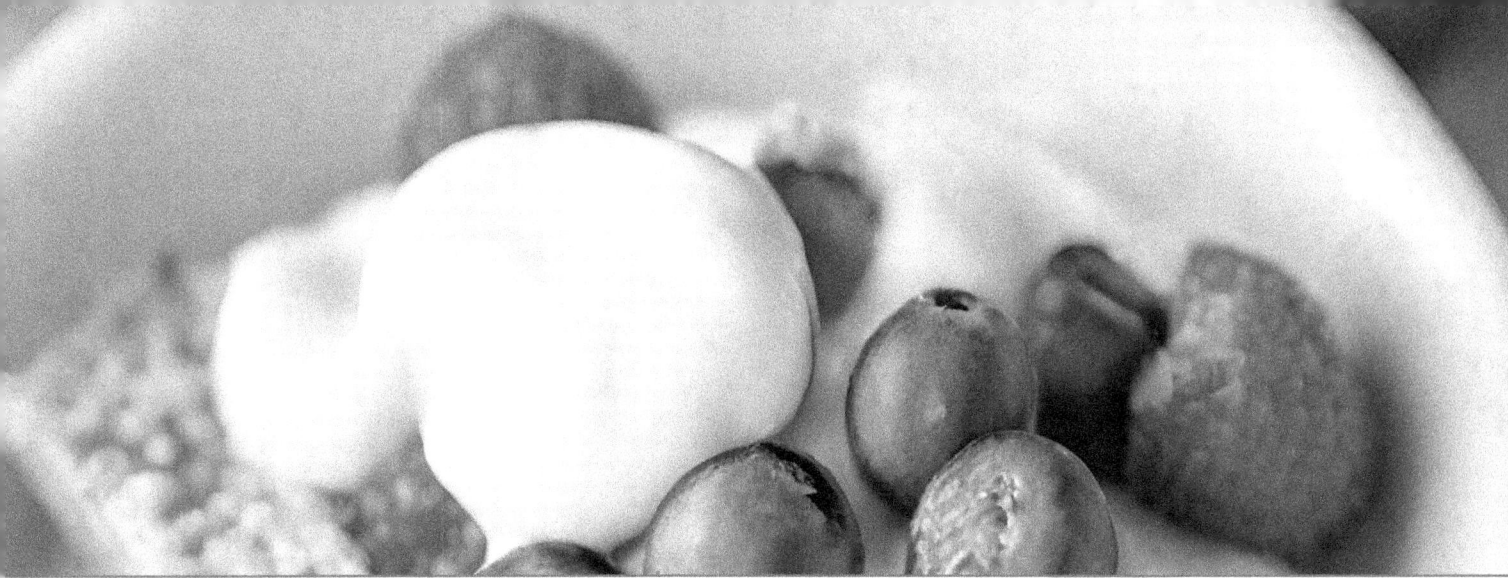

33. Greek Yogurt Parfait

Benefits: This snack offers protein and probiotics, beneficial for digestive health.

Servings: 1   **Prep/Cook Time: 5 Minutes**

Ingredients:

- 1/2 cup plain Greek yogurt
- 1/4 cup low-potassium granola
- 1/4 cup sliced bananas
- 1 tablespoon honey (optional)

Cooking Instructions:

1. In a glass or bowl, layer Greek yogurt, low-potassium granola, and sliced bananas.
2. Drizzle with honey if desired.

Nutritional Information (per serving): Approximately 220 calories, 11g protein, 38g carbohydrates, 3g fiber, 14g sugar, 3g fat, 70mg sodium.

Modification Tip: For lower potassium, reduce the portion of bananas or choose lower-potassium fruits.

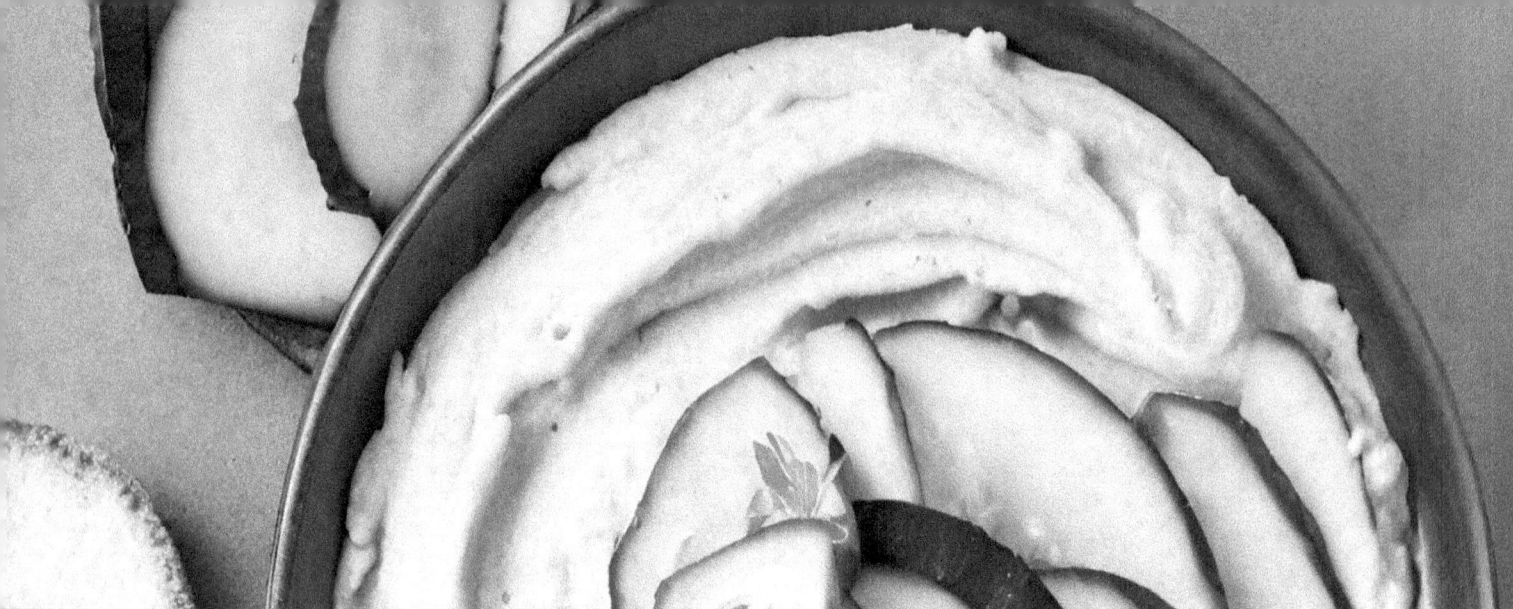

34. Hummus with Cucumber Slices

Benefits: These sweet potato fries are a tasty and low-potassium snack.

Servings: 1

Prep/Cook Time: 5 Minutes

Ingredients:

- 1/4 cup hummus
- 1 small cucumber, sliced

Cooking Instructions:

1. Slice the cucumber into thin rounds.
2. Dip the cucumber slices in hummus and enjoy.

Nutritional Information (per serving): Approximately 150 calories, 6g protein, 15g carbohydrates, 5g fiber, 3g sugar, 8g fat, 100mg sodium.

Modification Tip: For lower sodium, choose low-sodium hummus. To reduce potassium, opt for celery or bell pepper slices instead of cucumber.

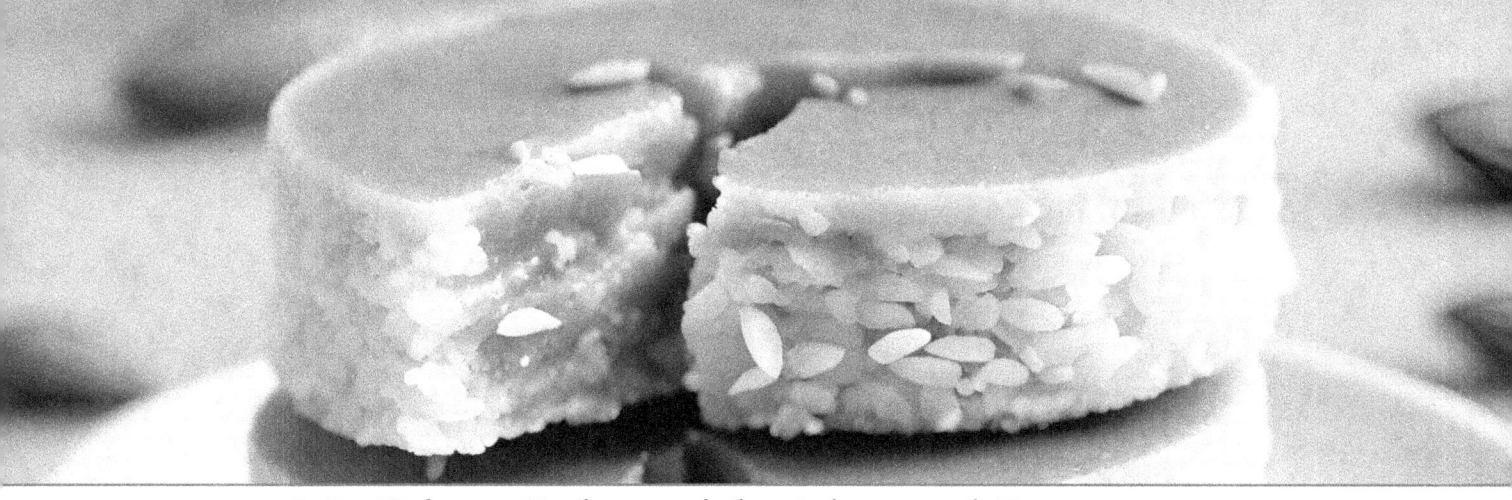

35. Rice Cake with Almond Butter

Benefits: This snack provides protein and healthy fats, and is low in phosphorus and potassium.

Servings: 1   **Prep/Cook Time: 5 Minutes**

Ingredients:

- 1 rice cake
- 2 tablespoons almond butter
- 1/2 small banana, sliced
- 1 teaspoon honey (optional)

Cooking Instructions:

1. Spread almond butter on the rice cake.
2. Top with banana slices and drizzle with honey if desired.

Nutritional Information (per serving): Approximately 190 calories, 4g protein, 20g carbohydrates, 3g fiber, 9g sugar, 12g fat, 0mg sodium.

Modification Tip: For lower sodium, use a rice cake with no added salt. To reduce potassium, omit the banana or choose a lower-potassium fruit.

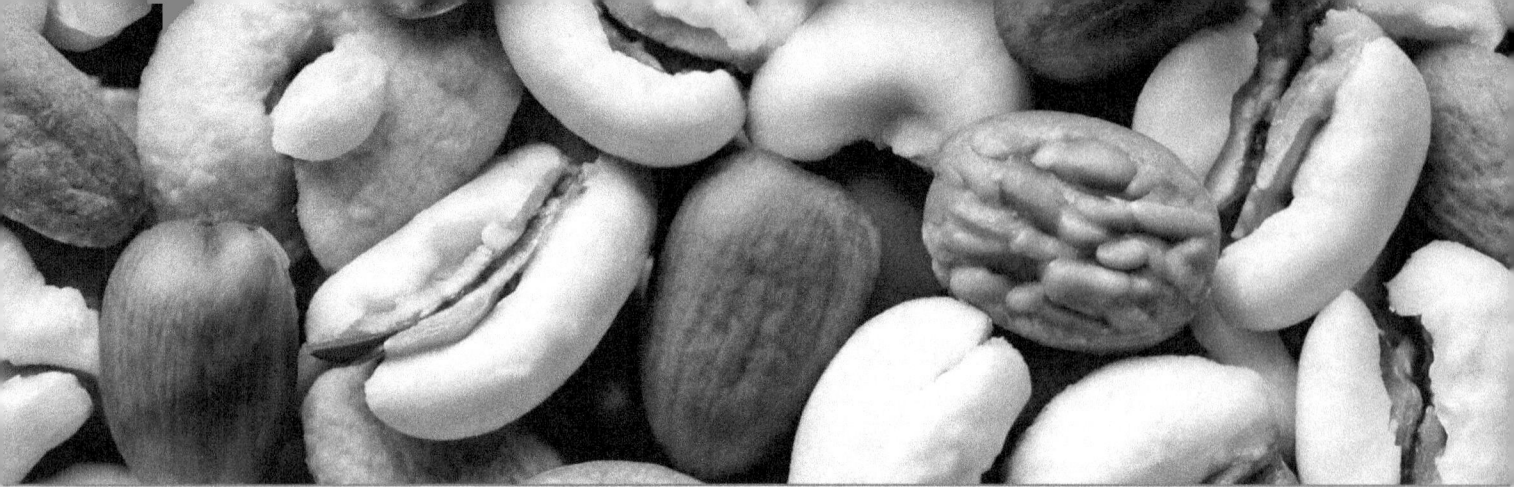

36. Mixed Nuts

Benefits: A handful of mixed nuts provides healthy fats and protein.

Servings: 1

Ingredients:

- 1 small handful of unsalted mixed nuts (e.g., almonds, walnuts, cashews)

Prep/Cook Time: 1 Minutes

Cooking Instructions:

1. Simply grab a small handful of mixed nuts and enjoy as a quick and healthy snack.

Nutritional Information (per serving): Approximately 180 calories, 6g protein, 5g carbohydrates, 2g fiber, 1g sugar, 16g fat, minimal sodium.

Modification Tip: Opt for unsalted or low-sodium mixed nuts to reduce sodium content.

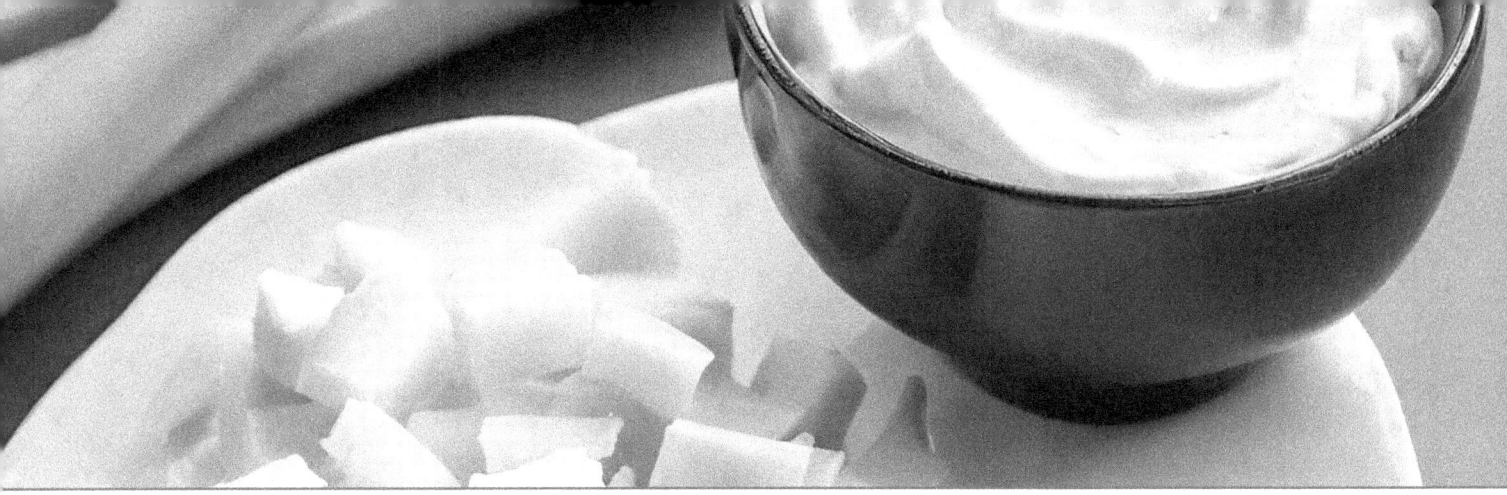

37. Celery and Cream Cheese

Benefits: A classic combination that's low in potassium and phosphorus.

Servings: 1

Ingredients:

- 2 celery stalks, cut into sticks
- 2 tablespoons low-fat cream cheese

Prep/Cook Time: 5 Minutes

Cooking Instructions:

1. Fill the celery sticks with low-fat cream cheese.
2. Enjoy this simple and crunchy snack.

Nutritional Information (per serving): Approximately 80 calories, 2g protein, 4g carbohydrates, 1g fiber, 3g sugar, 6g fat, 100mg sodium.

Modification Tip: Choose low-sodium cream cheese to further reduce sodium content.

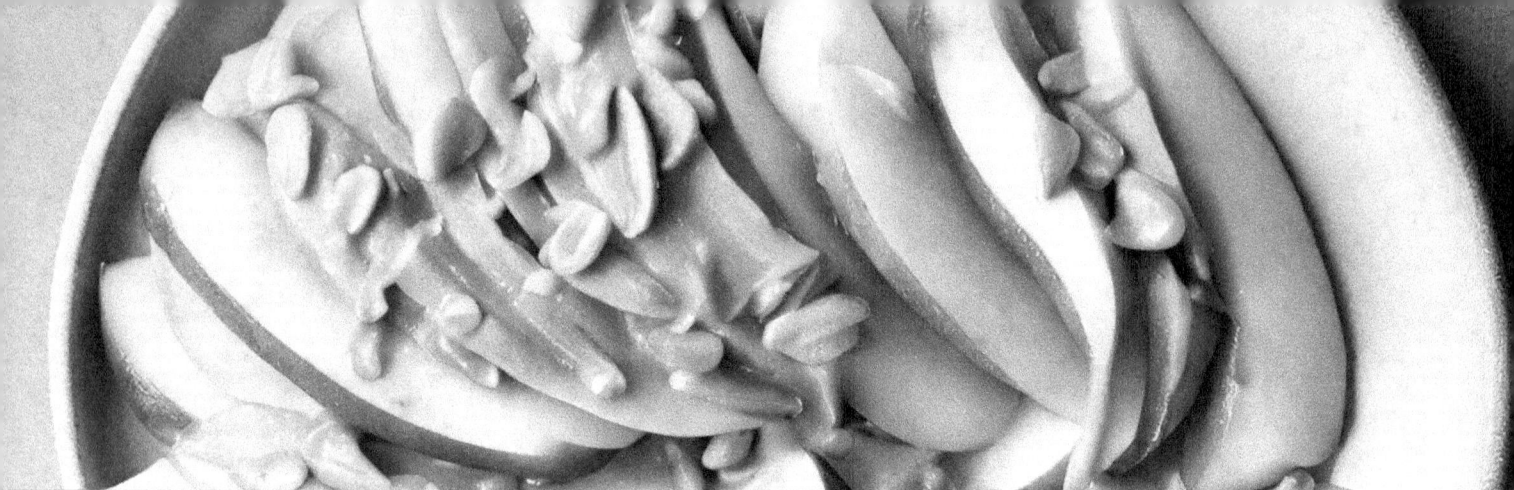

38. Sliced Apples with Peanut Butter

Benefits: Apples provide fiber and peanut butter offers protein.

Servings: 1   **Prep/Cook Time: 5 Minutes**

Ingredients:

- 1 small apple, sliced
- 2 tablespoons peanut butter

Cooking Instructions:

1. Slice the apple into wedges.
2. Dip the apple slices in peanut butter and enjoy.

Nutritional Information (per serving): Approximately 260 calories, 7g protein, 29g carbohydrates, 6g fiber, 19g sugar, 14g fat, 140mg sodium.

Modification Tip: For lower sodium, choose natural peanut butter with no added salt.

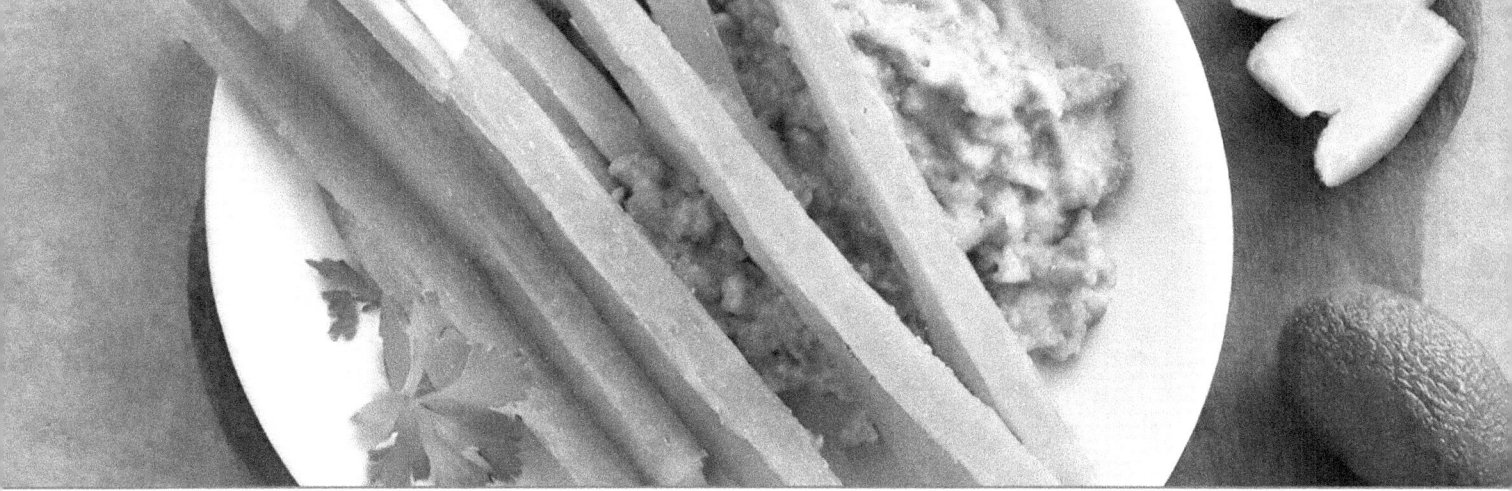

39. Carrot Sticks with Guacamole

Benefits: Carrots are low in potassium and phosphorus, while guacamole offers healthy fats.

Servings: 1　　　　**Prep/Cook Time: 10 Minutes**

Ingredients:

- 2 medium carrots, cut into sticks
- 1/4 cup guacamole

Cooking Instructions:

3. Cut the carrots into stick shapes.
4. Dip the carrot sticks in guacamole and enjoy.

Nutritional Information (per serving): Approximately 150 calories, 2g protein, 13g carbohydrates, 6g fiber, 4g sugar, 11g fat, 100mg sodium.

Modification Tip: For lower sodium, choose a low-sodium guacamole or make your own with minimal salt. To reduce potassium, consume a smaller portion of guacamole.

1.5 Soup And Salad

40. *Chicken and Rice Soup*

41. *Cucumber and Tomato Salad*

42. *Minestrone Soup*

43. *Spinach and Strawberry Salad*

44. *Tuna Salad*

45. *Potato Leek Soup*

46. *Quinoa and Black Bean Salad*

47. *Broccoli and Cauliflower Soup*

48. *Waldorf Salad*

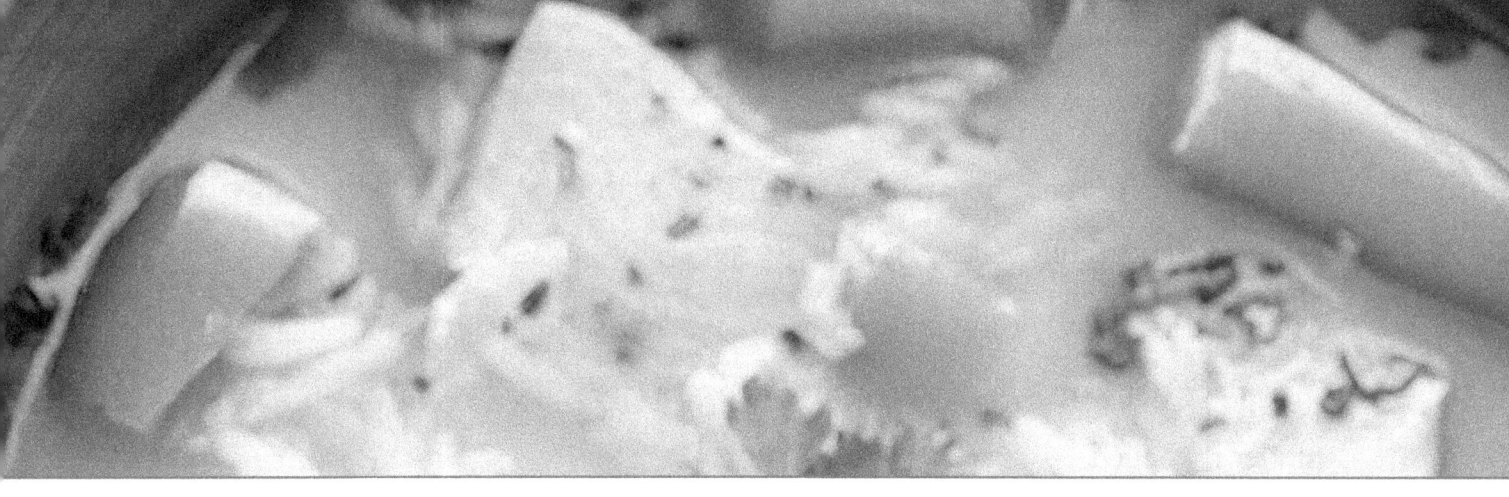

40. Chicken and Rice Soup

Benefits: This soup provides lean protein and is low in potassium and phosphorus.

Servings: 4   **Prep/Cook Time: 30 Minutes**

Ingredients:

- 2 boneless, skinless chicken breasts (about 4-6 ounces each)
- 1/2 cup white rice
- 1/2 cup carrots, diced
- 1/2 cup celery, diced
- 1/2 cup onion, chopped
- 1 clove garlic, minced
- 8 cups low-sodium chicken broth
- Salt and pepper to taste

Cooking Instructions:

1. In a large pot, bring the chicken broth to a boil.
2. Add chicken breasts and simmer until cooked through. Remove the chicken and shred it.
3. In the same pot, add rice, carrots, celery, onion, and garlic. Cook until vegetables are tender.
4. Return shredded chicken to the pot and season with salt and pepper.

Nutritional Information (per serving): Approximately 200 calories, 20g protein, 20g carbohydrates, 1g fiber, 1g sugar, 3g fat, 120mg sodium.

Modification Tip: For lower sodium, choose low-sodium chicken broth. To reduce potassium, reduce the portion of carrots and use a phosphate binder if needed.

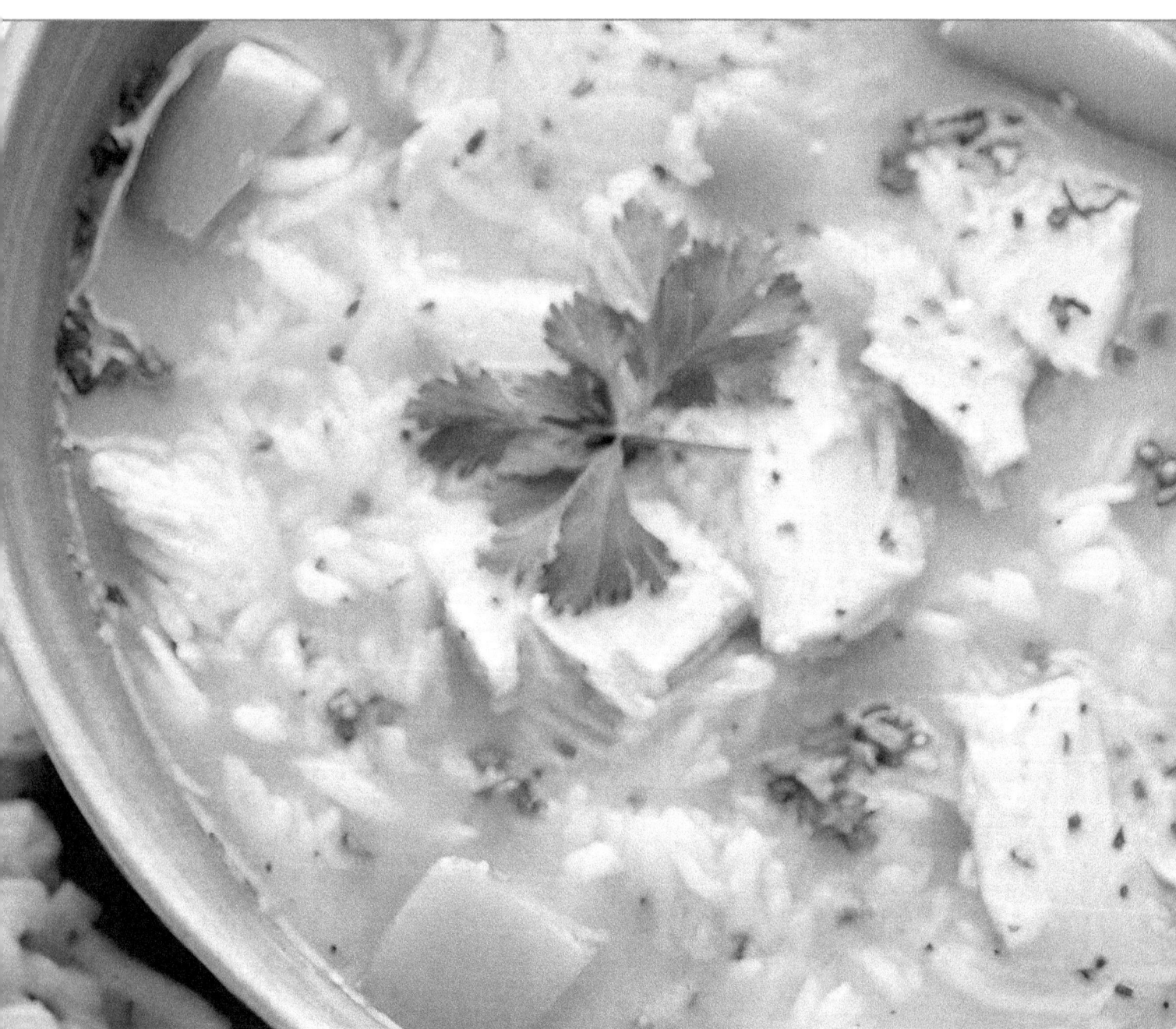

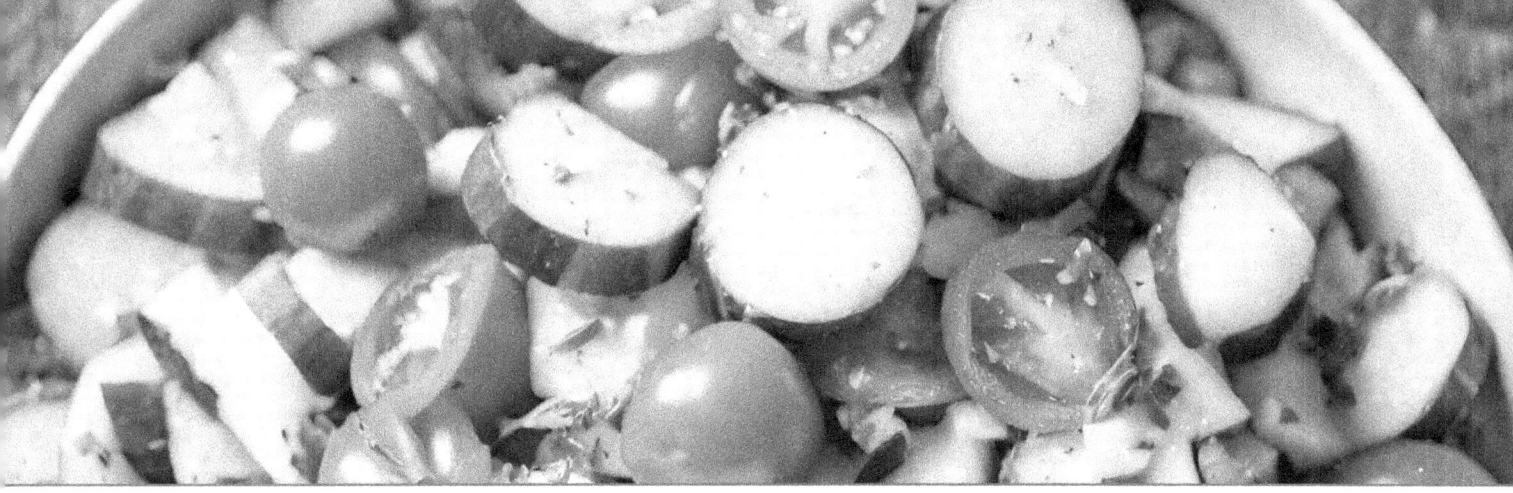

41. Cucumber and Tomato Salad

Benefits: This salad is low in potassium and phosphorus and provides hydration.

Servings: 4

Prep/Cook Time: 30 Minutes

Ingredients:

- 2 cucumbers, sliced
- 2 large tomatoes, diced
- 1/4 cup red onion, finely chopped
- 2 tablespoons fresh basil, chopped
- 2 tablespoons balsamic vinegar
- Salt and pepper to taste

Cooking Instructions:

1. In a bowl, combine sliced cucumbers, diced tomatoes, chopped red onion, and fresh basil.
2. Drizzle balsamic vinegar over the salad and season with salt and pepper.

Nutritional Information (per serving): Approximately 60 calories, 2g protein, 14g carbohydrates, 3g fiber, 7g sugar, 0g fat, 20mg sodium.

Modification Tip: To further reduce sodium, use a salt substitute or omit salt. If potassium is a concern, reduce the portion of tomatoes.

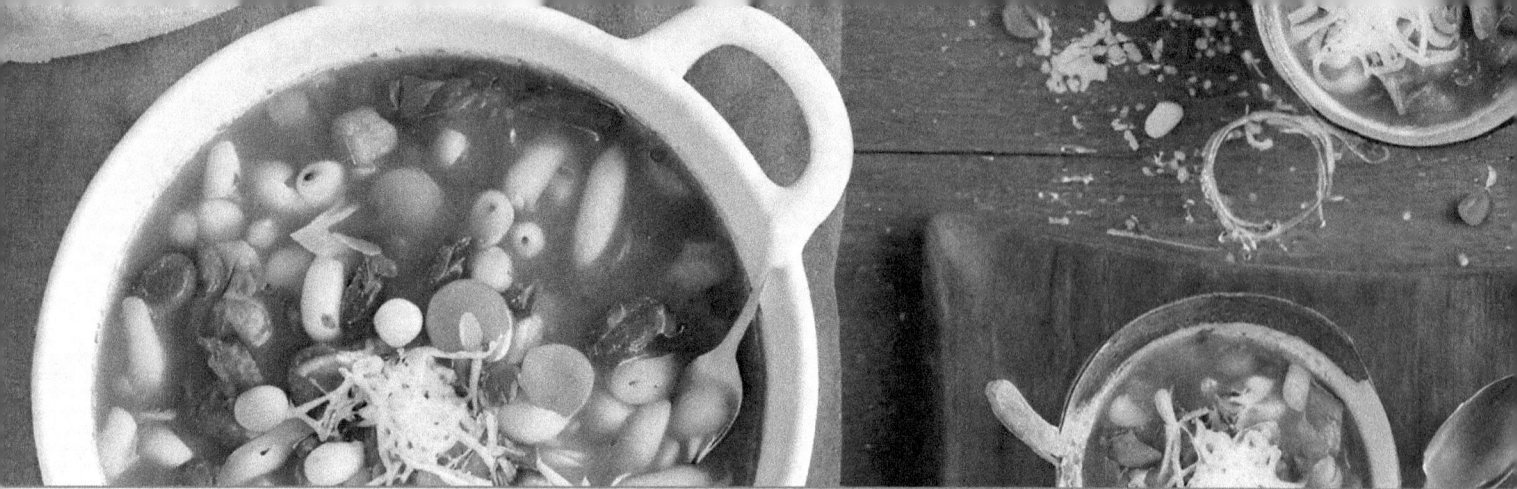

42. Minestrone Soup

Benefits: This soup provides lean protein and is low in potassium and phosphorus.

Servings: 4

Prep/Cook Time: 30 Minutes

Ingredients:

- 1 cup low-sodium vegetable broth
- 1/2 cup zucchini, diced
- 1/2 cup carrots, diced
- 1/2 cup celery, diced
- 1/2 cup green beans, cut into 1-inch pieces
- 1/2 cup onion, chopped
- 1 clove garlic, minced
- 1 can (14 ounces) low-sodium diced tomatoes

Cooking Instructions:

1. In a large pot, heat vegetable broth over medium heat.
2. Add zucchini, carrots, celery, green beans, onion, and garlic. Cook until vegetables are tender.
3. Stir in diced tomatoes, kidney beans, white beans, green peas, and whole wheat pasta.
4. Simmer until the pasta is cooked.
5. Season with fresh basil, salt, and pepper.

Ingredients:

- 1/2 cup low-sodium kidney beans, drained and rinsed
- 1/2 cup low-sodium white beans, drained and rinsed
- 1/2 cup low-sodium green peas
- 1/2 cup whole wheat pasta
- 1/4 cup fresh basil, chopped
- Salt and pepper to taste

Nutritional Information (per serving): Approximately 200 calories, 9g protein, 40g carbohydrates, 10g fiber, 8g sugar, 1g fat, 50mg sodium.

Modification Tip: To reduce sodium further, use a salt substitute and choose low-sodium beans and pasta. For lower potassium, reduce the portion of beans.

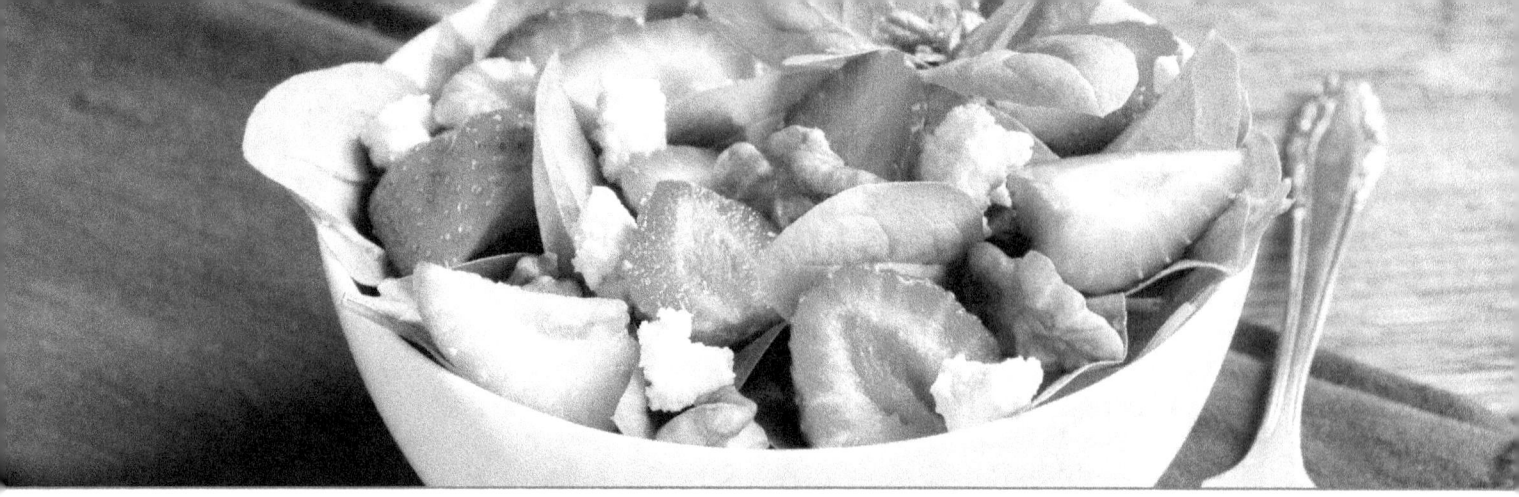

43. Spinach and Strawberry Salad

Benefits: This salad is rich in vitamins and antioxidants, and it is low in potassium and phosphorus.

Servings: 2

Prep/Cook Time: 10 Minutes

Ingredients:

- 4 cups fresh spinach leaves
- 1 cup fresh strawberries, sliced
- 1/4 cup red onion, finely chopped
- 1/4 cup feta cheese, crumbled
- 2 tablespoons balsamic vinaigrette
- Salt and pepper to taste

Cooking Instructions:

1. In a bowl, combine fresh spinach leaves, sliced strawberries, chopped red onion, and crumbled feta cheese.

2. Drizzle balsamic vinaigrette over the salad and season with salt and pepper.

Nutritional Information (per serving): Approximately 140 calories, 7g protein, 17g carbohydrates, 4g fiber, 8g sugar, 6g fat, 300mg sodium.

Modification Tip: For lower sodium, use a salt substitute or omit salt. If potassium is a concern, reduce the portion of strawberries.

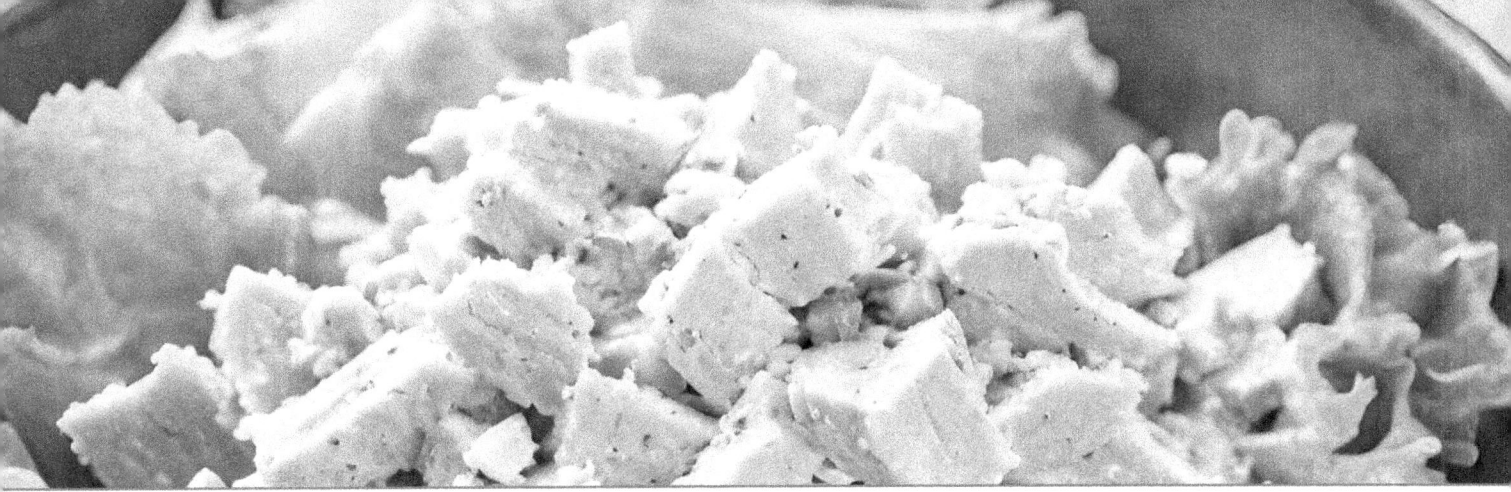

44. Tuna Salad

Benefits: This salad is a good source of protein and is low in potassium and phosphorus.

Servings: 2

Prep/Cook Time: 10 Minutes

Ingredients:

- 1 can (5 ounces) low-sodium tuna, drained
- 1/4 cup red onion, finely chopped
- 1/4 cup celery, diced
- 1/4 cup low-fat mayonnaise
- 2 teaspoons Dijon mustard
- Salt and pepper to taste

Cooking Instructions:

1. In a bowl, combine drained tuna, chopped red onion, diced celery, low-fat mayonnaise, and Dijon mustard.
2. Season with salt and pepper.

Nutritional Information (per serving): Approximately 150 calories, 20g protein, 3g carbohydrates, 1g fiber, 2g sugar, 6g fat, 250mg sodium.

Modification Tip: For lower sodium, use a salt substitute and low-sodium mayonnaise. To reduce potassium, reduce the portion of celery.

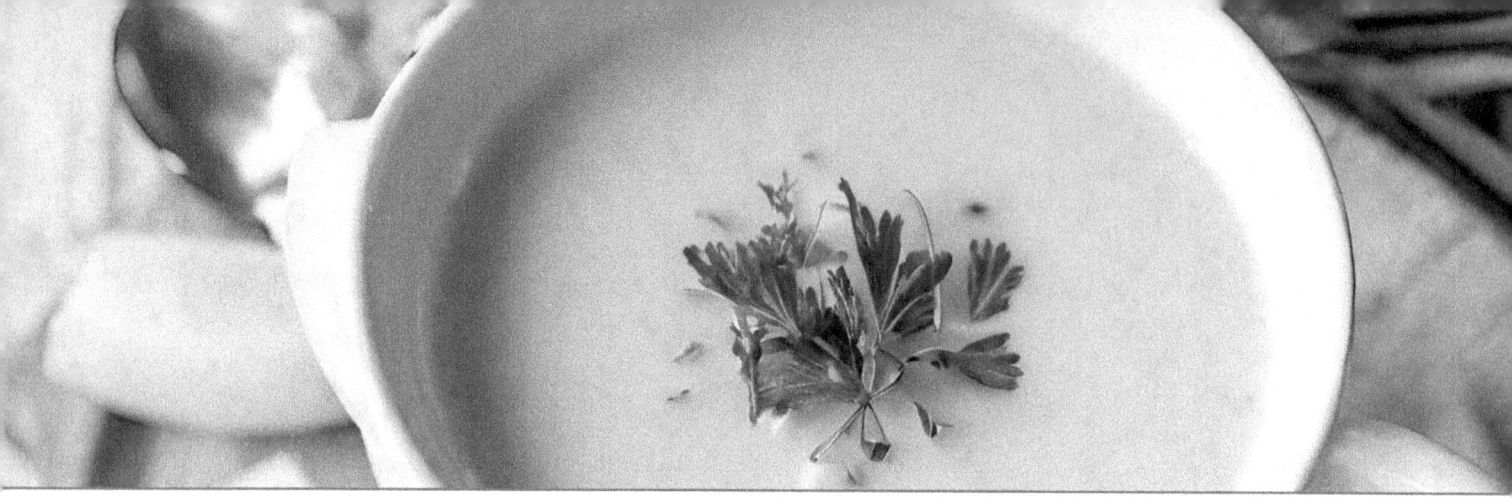

45. Potato Leek Soup

Benefits: This soup is creamy and comforting, yet low in potassium and phosphorus.

Servings: 4

Prep/Cook Time: 45 Minutes

Ingredients:

- 4 cups leeks, sliced (white and light green parts only)
- 2 cups potatoes, peeled and diced
- 4 cups low-sodium vegetable broth
- 1/2 cup low-fat sour cream
- 1/4 cup fresh chives, chopped
- Salt and pepper to taste.

Cooking Instructions:

1. In a large pot, combine leeks, potatoes, and vegetable broth.
2. Bring to a boil, then reduce heat and simmer for about 30-35 minutes, or until potatoes are tender.
3. Use an immersion blender or regular blender to puree the soup until smooth.
4. Stir in low-fat sour cream, fresh chives, salt, and pepper.

Nutritional Information (per serving): Approximately 160 calories, 3g protein, 35g carbohydrates, 3g fiber, 5g sugar, 1g fat, 100mg sodium.

Modification Tip: For lower sodium, choose low-sodium vegetable broth. To reduce potassium, reduce the portion of potatoes.

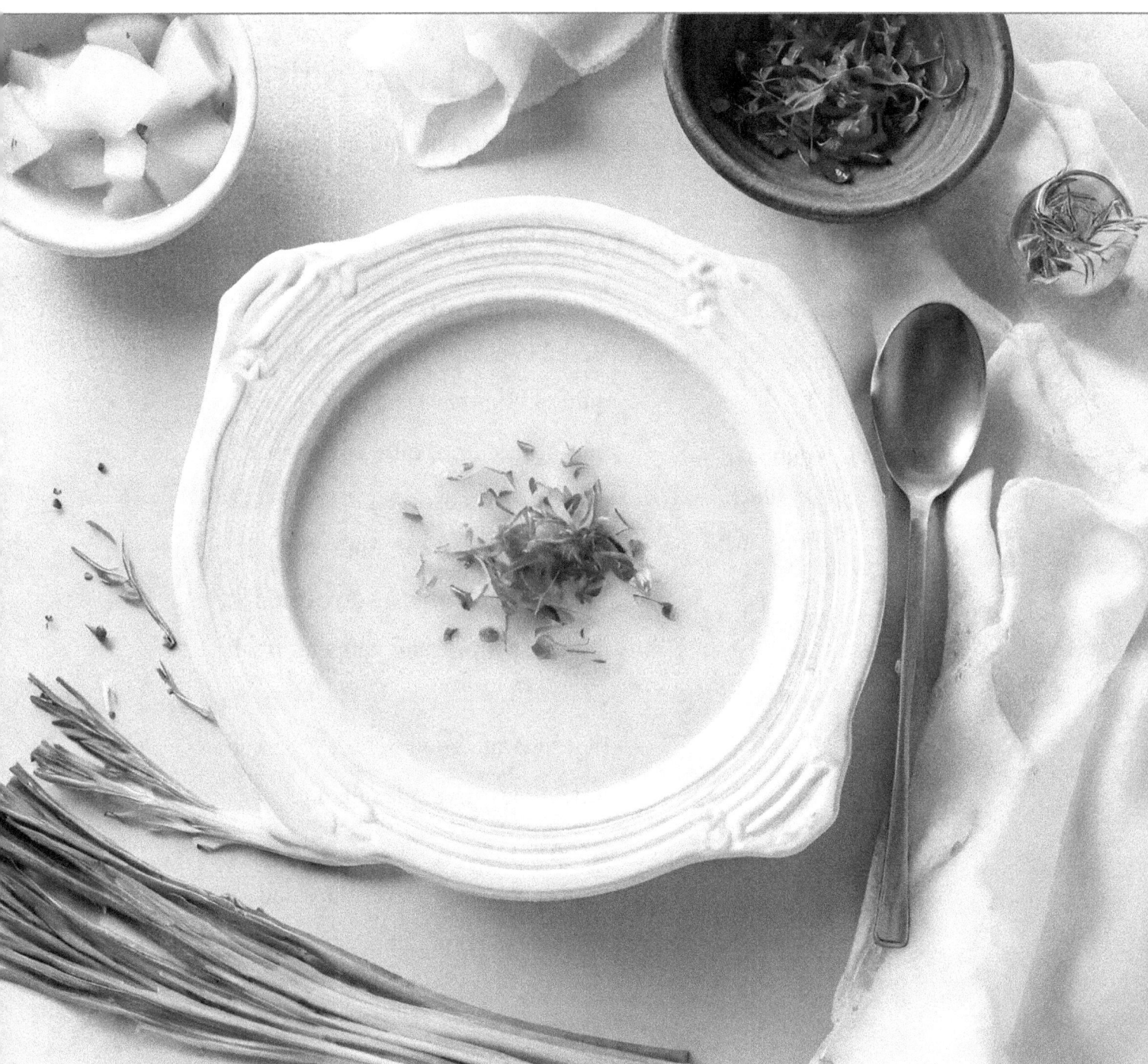

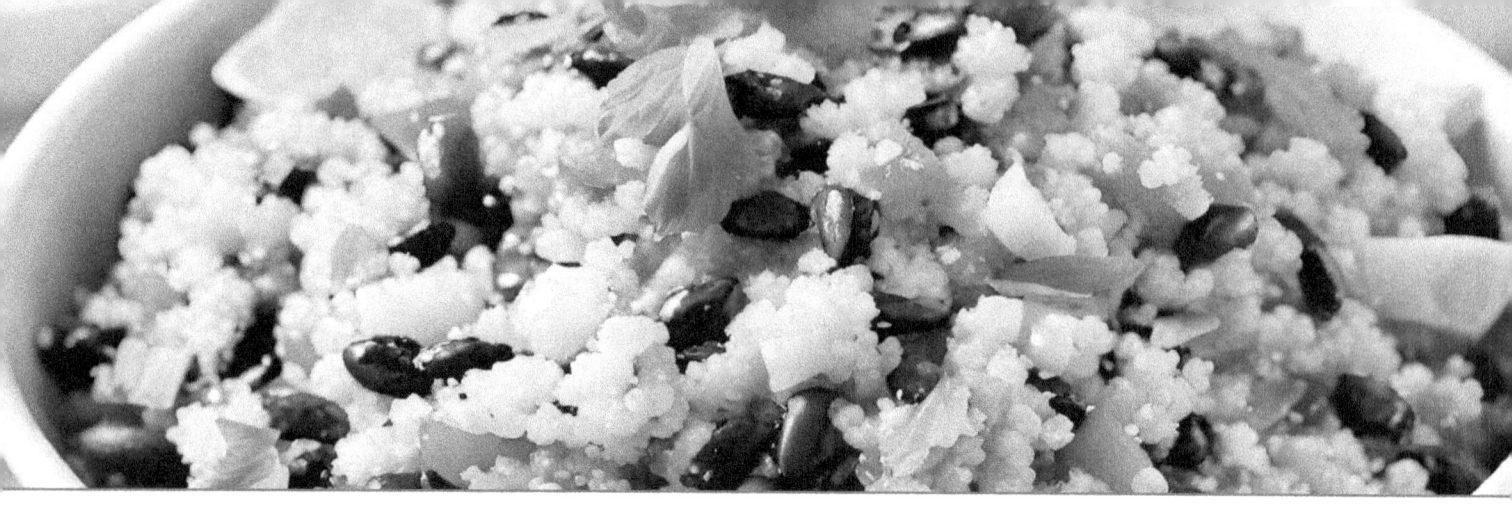

46. Quinoa and Black Bean Salad

Benefits: This salad provides plant-based protein and is low in potassium and phosphorus.

Servings: 4

Prep/Cook Time: 15 Minutes

Ingredients:

- 1 cup quinoa, rinsed
- 2 cups water
- 1 can (15 ounces) low-sodium black beans, drained and rinsed
- 1 cup corn (fresh, frozen, or canned, no salt added)
- 1/2 cup red bell pepper, diced
- 1/4 cup fresh cilantro, chopped
- 1/4 cup lime juice
- 2 tablespoons olive oil

Cooking Instructions:

1. Boil 2 cups of water and add quinoa. Simmer for about 15 minutes, or until quinoa is cooked and water is absorbed.
2. In a large bowl, combine cooked quinoa, black beans, corn, diced red bell pepper, and chopped fresh cilantro.
3. In a separate bowl, whisk together lime juice, olive oil, salt, and pepper.
4. Pour the dressing over the salad and toss to combine.

Ingredients:

- Salt and pepper to taste

Nutritional Information (per serving): Approximately 220 calories, 8g protein, 38g carbohydrates, 7g fiber, 4g sugar, 6g fat, 100mg sodium.

Modification Tip: For lower sodium, use a salt substitute and low-sodium black beans. To reduce potassium, reduce the portion of black beans.

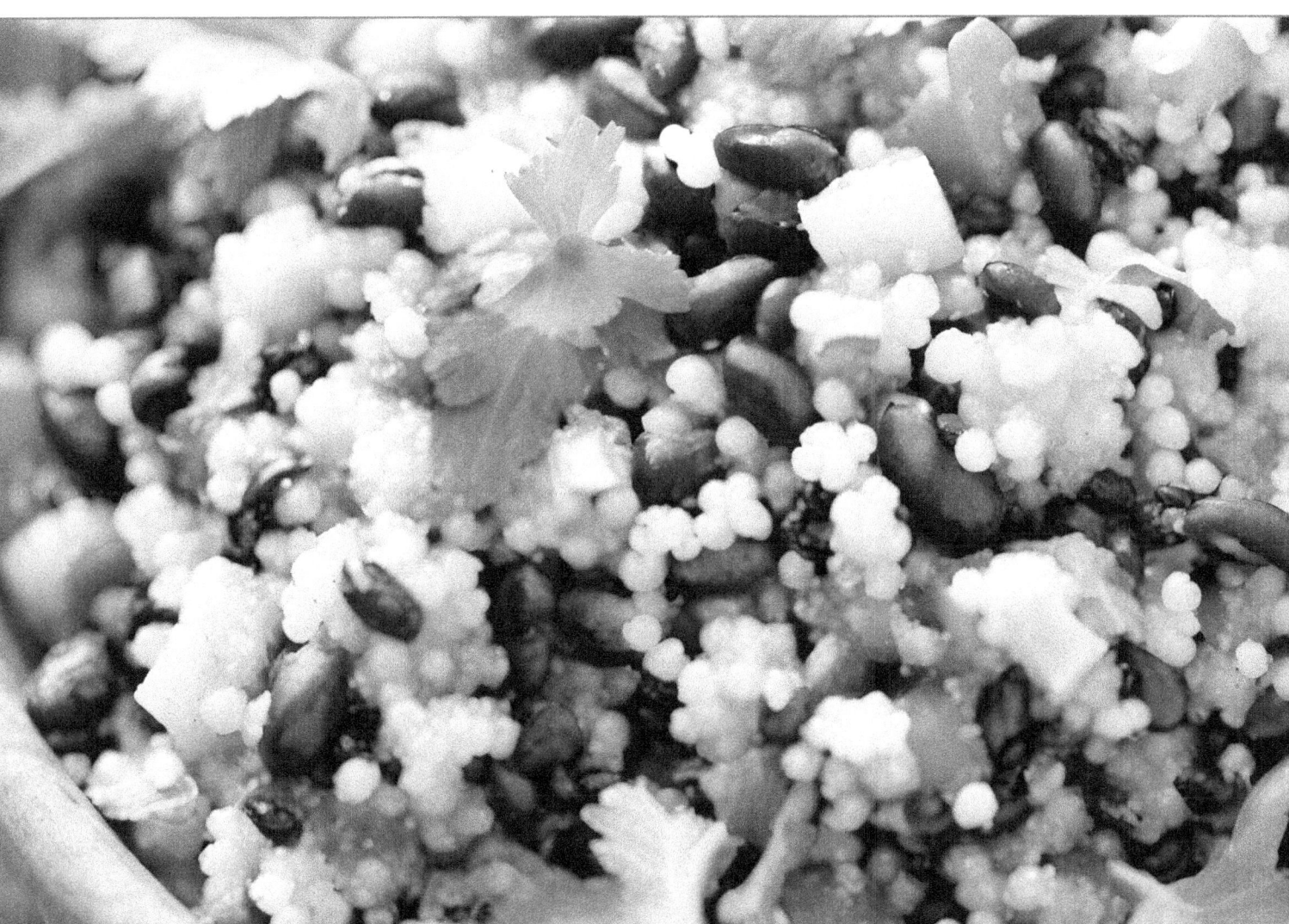

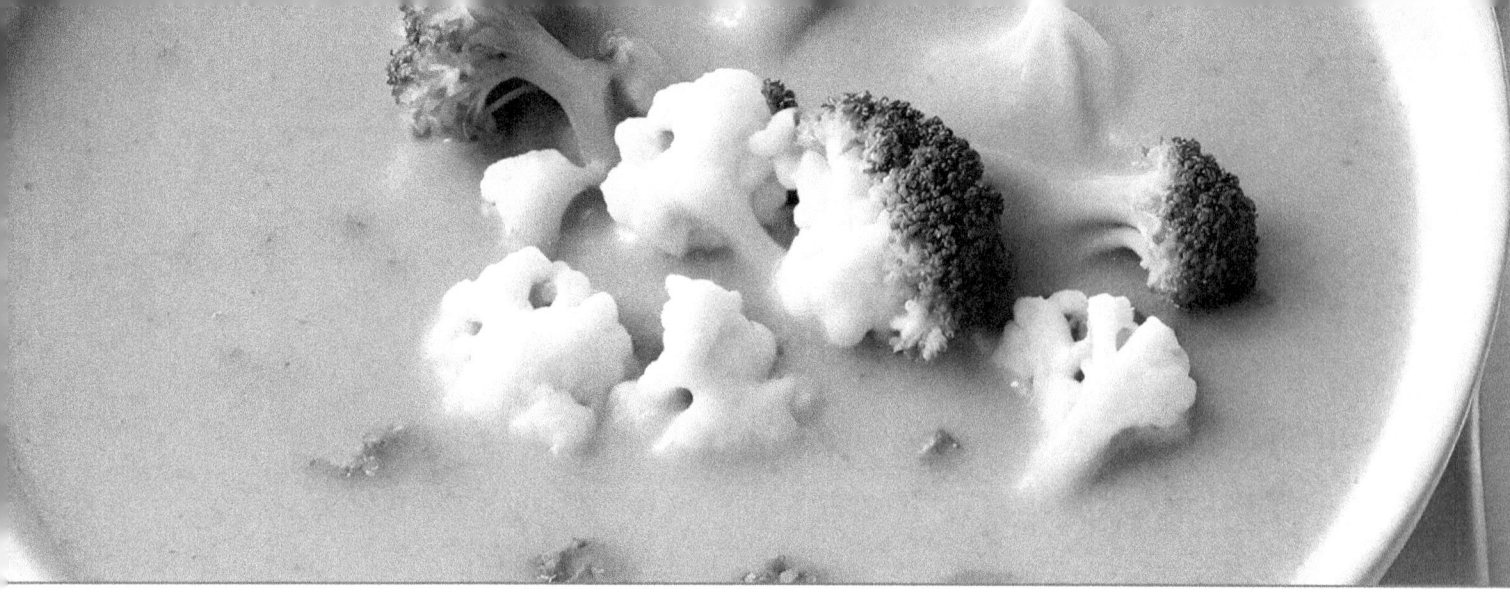

47. Broccoli and Cauliflower Soup

Benefits: This soup is rich in fiber and low in potassium and phosphorus.

Servings: 4

Ingredients:

- 2 cups broccoli, chopped
- 2 cups cauliflower, chopped
- 1/2 cup onion, chopped
- 2 cloves garlic, minced
- 4 cups low-sodium vegetable broth
- 1/2 cup low-fat plain yogurt
- Salt and pepper to taste

Prep/Cook Time: 30 Minutes

Cooking Instructions:

1. In a large pot, combine broccoli, cauliflower, onion, garlic, and vegetable broth.
2. Bring to a boil, then reduce heat and simmer for about 20-25 minutes, or until vegetables are tender.
3. Use an immersion blender or regular blender to puree the soup until smooth.
4. Stir in low-fat plain yogurt, salt, and pepper.

Nutritional Information (per serving): Approximately 100 calories, 5g protein, 18g carbohydrates, 5g fiber, 6g sugar, 1g fat, 50mg sodium.

Modification Tip: For lower sodium, choose low-sodium vegetable broth. To reduce potassium, reduce the portion of broccoli and cauliflower.

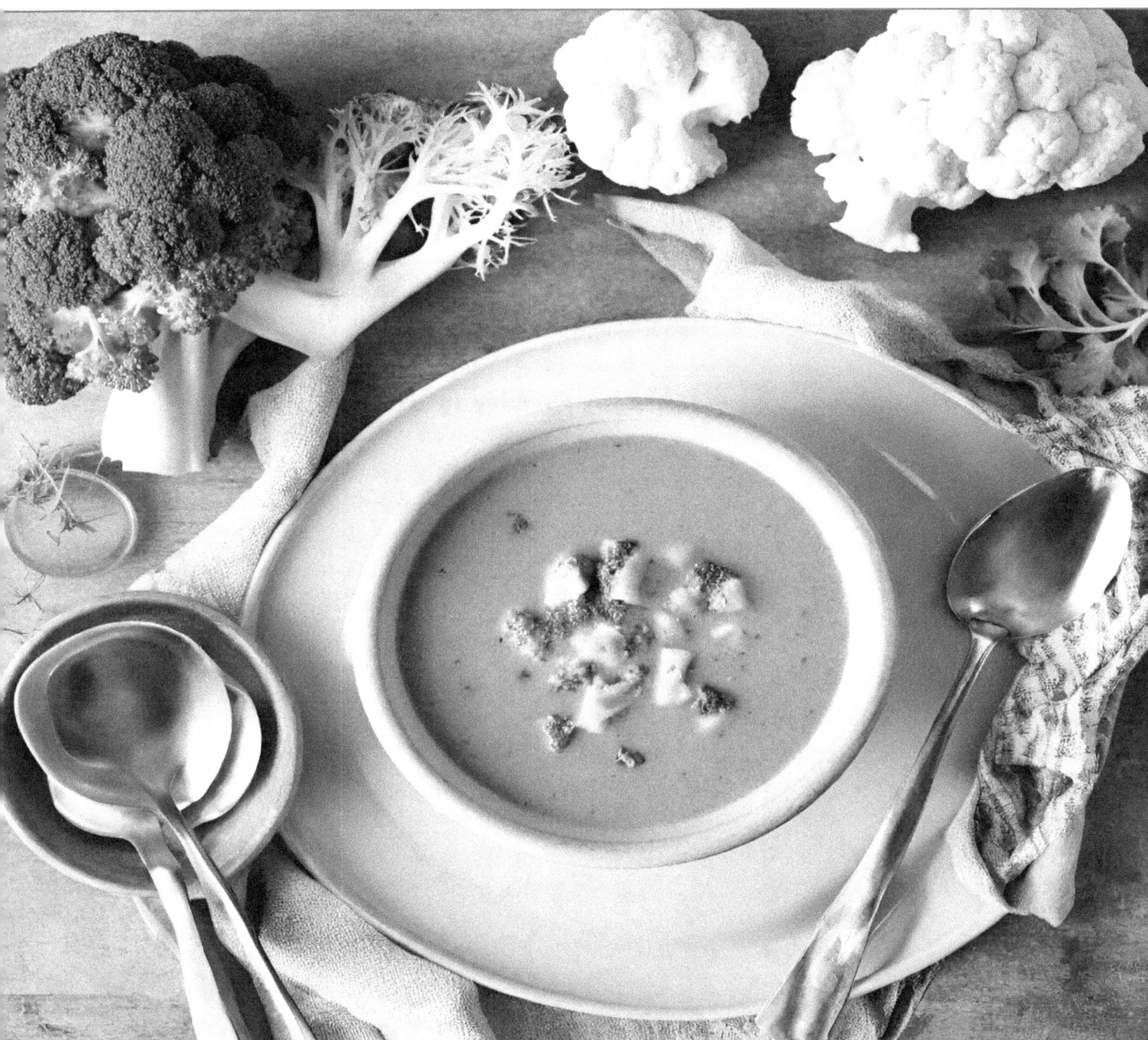

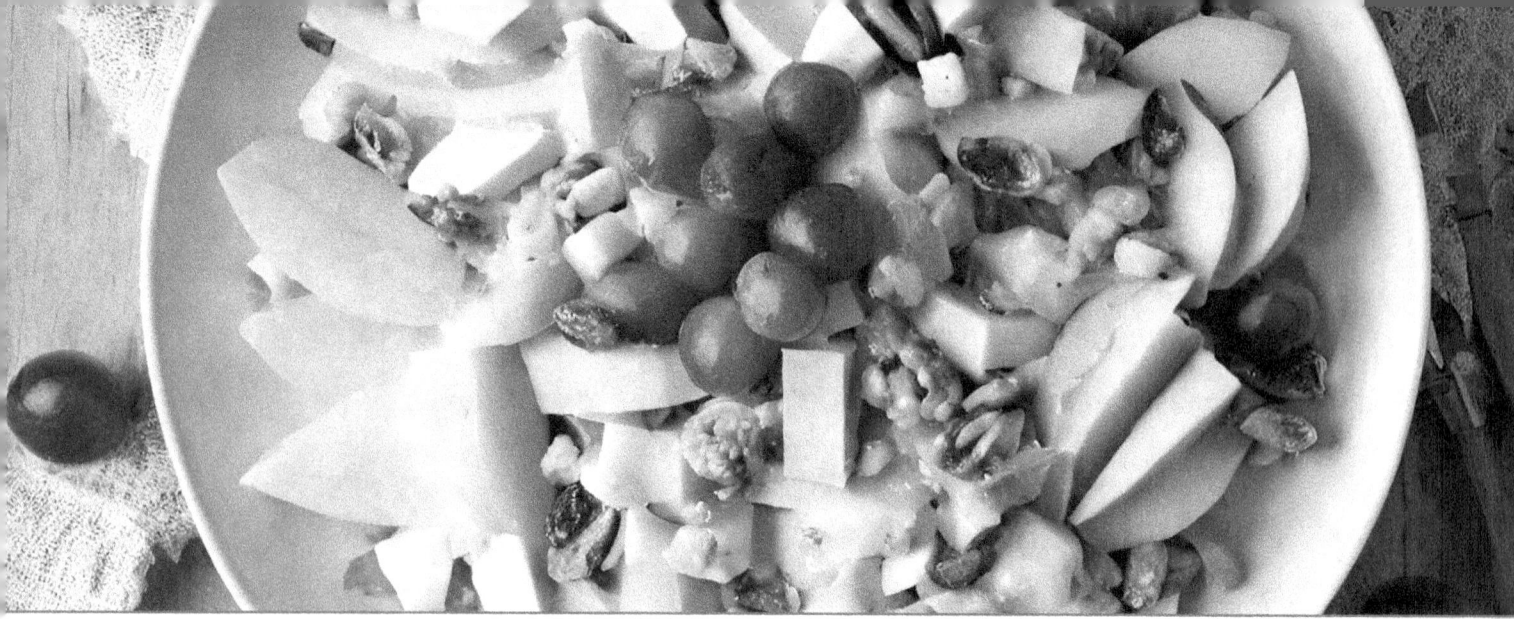

48. Waldorf Salad

Benefits: This soup is rich in fiber and low in potassium and phosphorus.

Servings: 4

Prep/Cook Time: 30 Minutes

Ingredients:

- 2 cups fresh apples, diced
- 1/2 cup celery, diced
- 1/4 cup walnuts, chopped
- 1/4 cup low-fat mayonnaise
- 1 tablespoon lemon juice
- Salt and pepper to taste

Cooking Instructions:

1. In a bowl, combine diced apples, diced celery, and chopped walnuts.

2. In a separate bowl, whisk together low-fat mayonnaise, lemon juice, salt, and pepper.

3. Pour the dressing over the salad and toss to combine.

Nutritional Information (per serving): Approximately 190 calories, 2g protein, 21g carbohydrates, 4g fiber, 16g sugar, 11g fat, 150mg sodium.

Modification Tip: For lower sodium, use a salt substitute and low-sodium mayonnaise. To reduce potassium, reduce the portion of apples and walnuts.

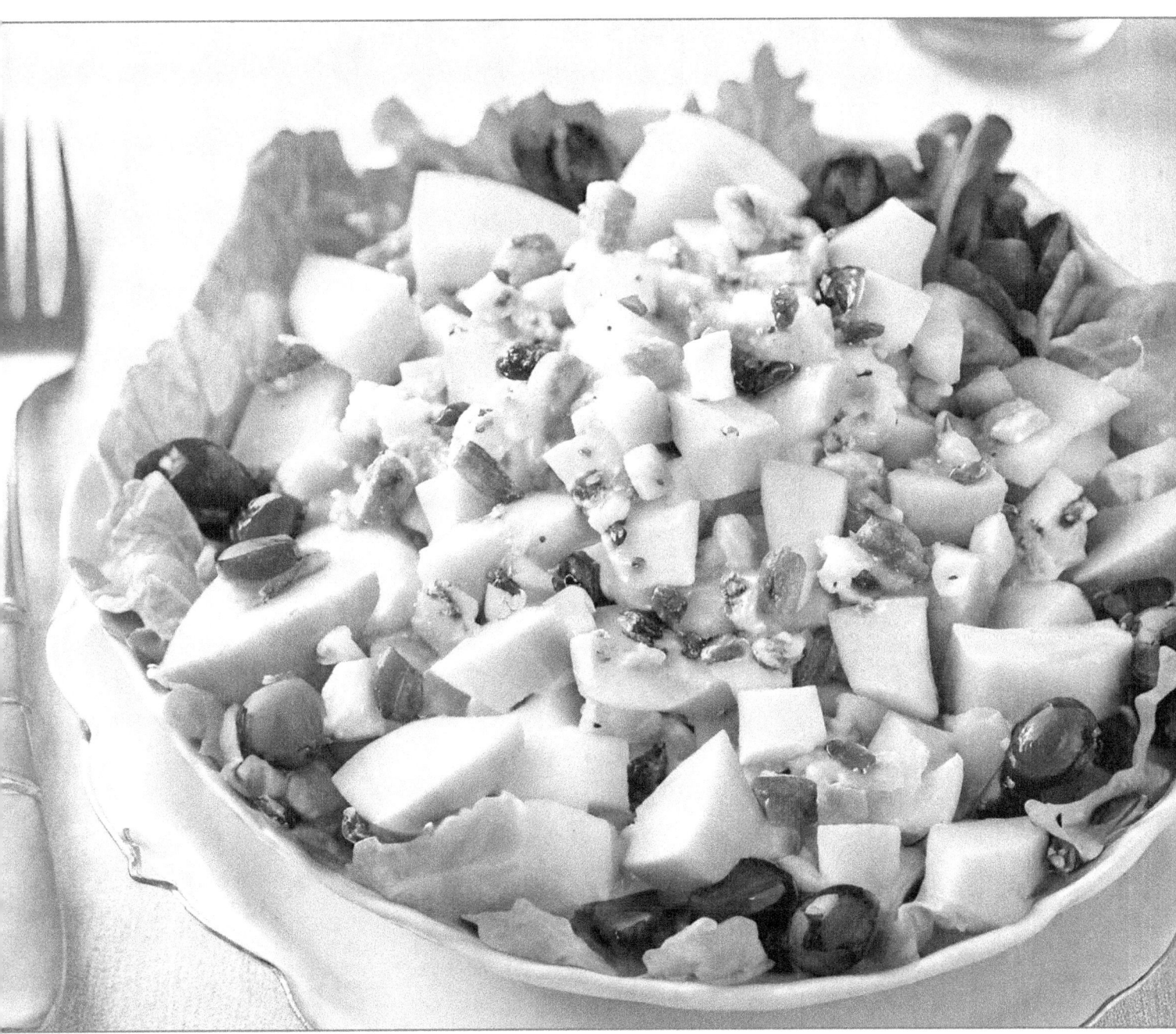

1.6 Dessert

49. Berry Parfait

50. Rice Pudding

51. Poached Pears

52. Pumpkin Pie Mousse

53. Banana Ice Cream

54. Almond Rice Cakes

55. Apple Crisp

56. Chocolate Avocado Pudding

57. Lemon Sorbet

58. Watermelon Granita

59. Baked Apples with Cinnamon and Walnuts

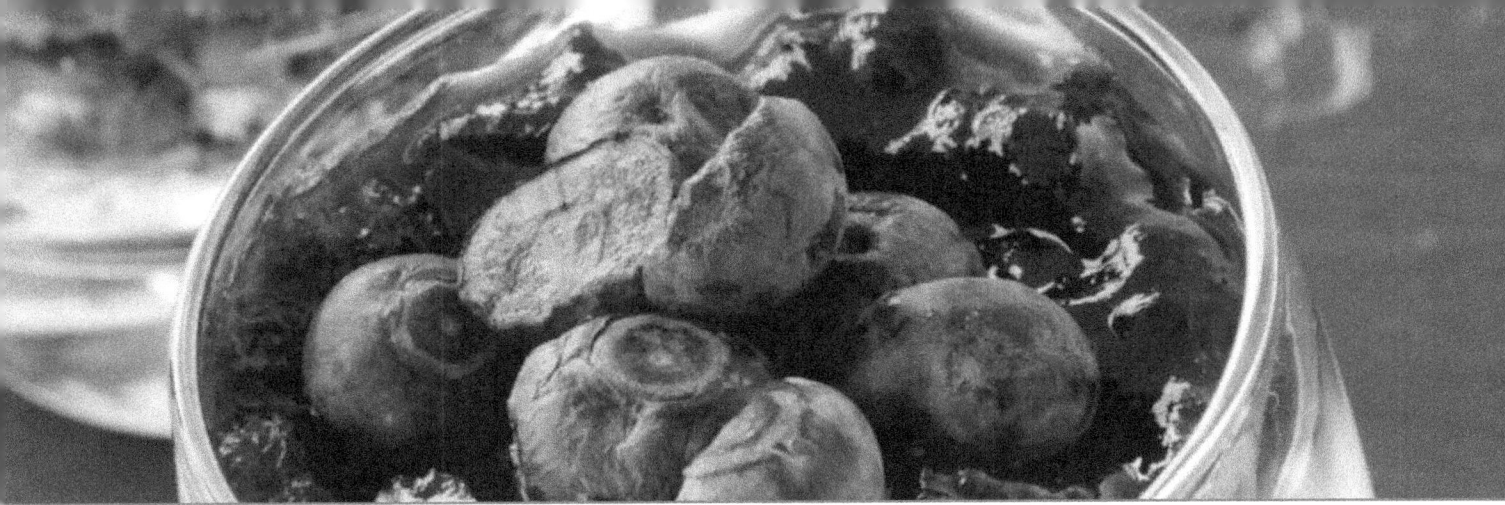

49. Berry Parfait

Benefits: This dessert is rich in antioxidants and low in potassium and phosphorus.

Servings: 2

Prep/Cook Time: 10 Minutes

Ingredients:

- 1 cup low-fat vanilla yogurt
- 1 cup mixed berries (e.g., strawberries, blueberries)
- 1/4 cup low-potassium granola
- Fresh mint leaves for garnish.

Cooking Instructions:

1. In a glass, layer low-fat vanilla yogurt, mixed berries, and low-potassium granola.
2. Repeat the layers, and garnish with fresh mint leaves.

Nutritional Information (per serving): Approximately 150 calories, 6g protein, 30g carbohydrates, 4g fiber, 10g sugar, 1g fat, 70mg sodium.

Modification Tip: For lower potassium, reduce the portion of berries.

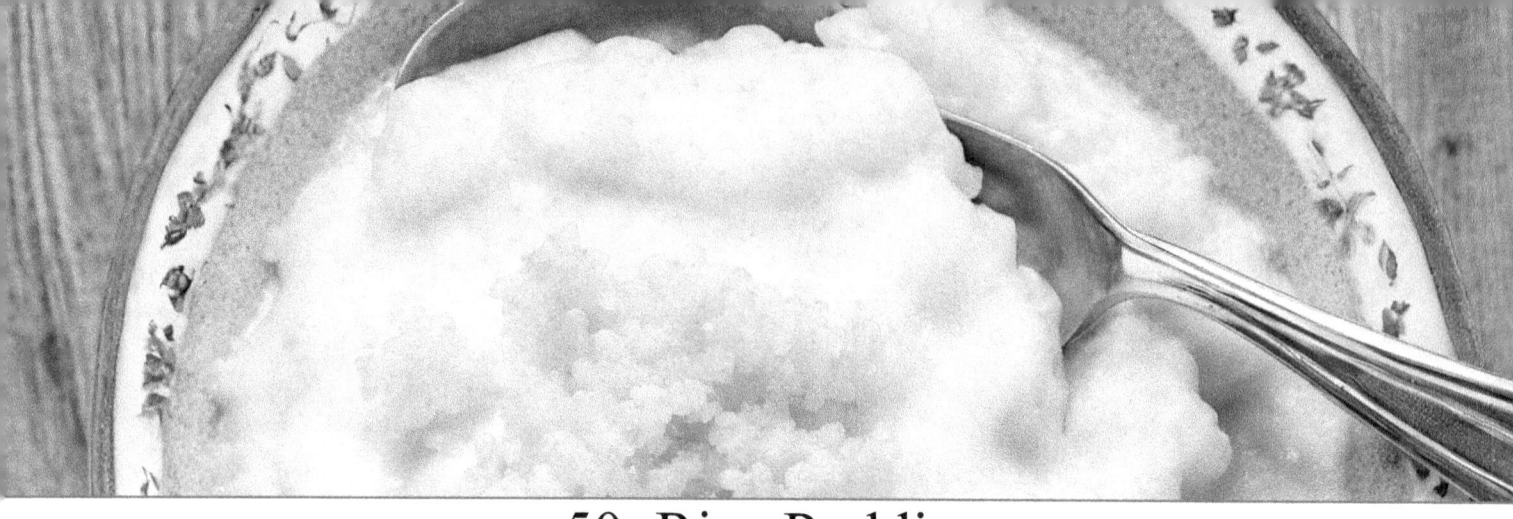

50. Rice Pudding

Benefits: This dessert is creamy and satisfying, yet low in potassium and phosphorus.

Servings: 4

Prep/Cook Time: 40 Minutes

Ingredients:

- 1/2 cup Arborio rice
- 2 cups low-fat milk
- 1/4 cup granulated sugar
- 1/2 teaspoon vanilla extract
- 1/4 teaspoon ground cinnamon
- A pinch of salt

Cooking Instructions:

1. In a saucepan, combine Arborio rice and low-fat milk.
2. Cook over medium heat, stirring occasionally, until the rice is tender and the mixture thickens.
3. Stir in granulated sugar, vanilla extract, ground cinnamon, and a pinch of salt.
4. Remove from heat and let it cool.

Nutritional Information (per serving): Approximately 180 calories, 4g protein, 36g carbohydrates, 1g fiber, 12g sugar, 2g fat, 70mg sodium.

Modification Tip: For lower sodium, use a salt substitute. To reduce potassium, consume a smaller portion.

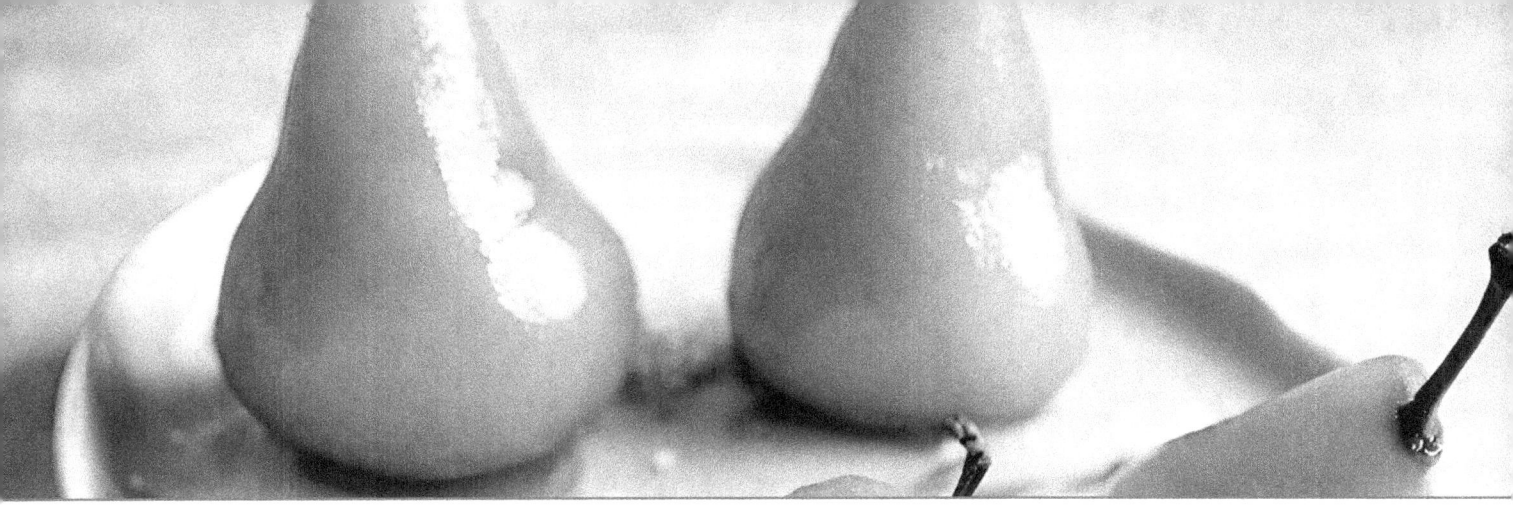

51. Poached Pears

Benefits: This dessert is a simple and elegant option, and it's low in potassium and phosphorus.

Servings: 4   **Prep/Cook Time: 20 Minutes**

Ingredients:

- 4 ripe pears, peeled and cored
- 2 cups water
- 1/2 cup granulated sugar
- 1 cinnamon stick
- 1 teaspoon lemon zest

Cooking Instructions:

1. In a large saucepan, combine water, granulated sugar, cinnamon stick, and lemon zest. Bring to a simmer.
2. Add peeled and cored pears to the simmering liquid and poach for about 10-15 minutes, or until they are tender.
3. Remove pears from the liquid and let them cool.
4. Serve with a drizzle of the poaching liquid.

Nutritional Information (per serving): Approximately 160 calories, 0g protein, 42g carbohydrates, 4g fiber, 32g sugar, 0g fat, 0mg sodium.

Modification Tip: To reduce potassium, consume a smaller portion of poached pears.

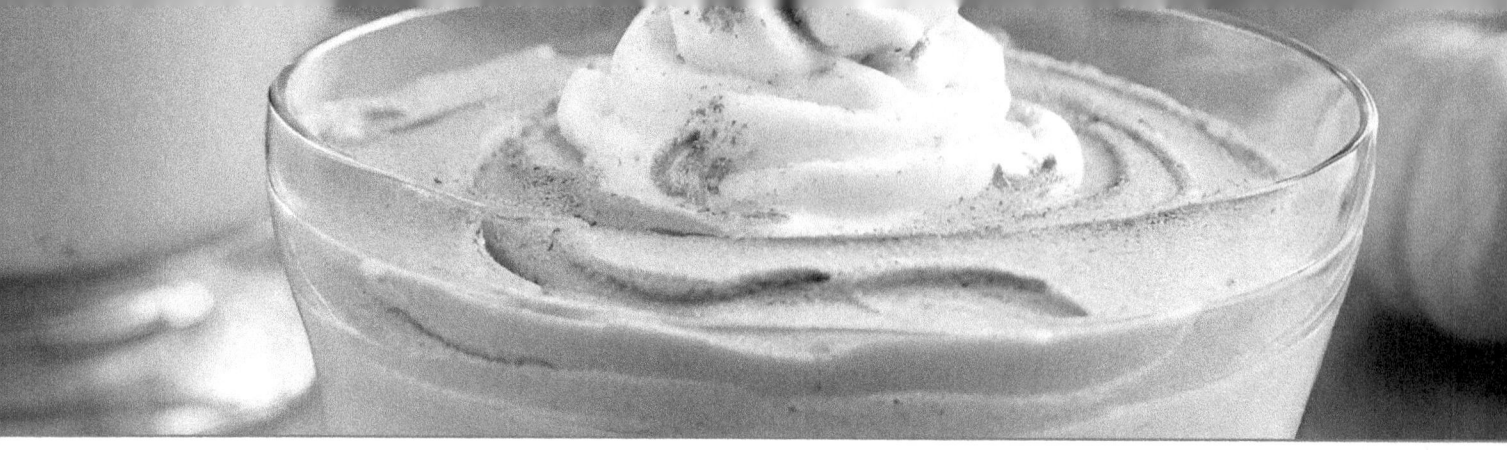

52. Pumpkin Pie Mousse

Benefits: This dessert offers a taste of pumpkin pie without the high potassium and phosphorus content.

Servings: 4

Prep/Cook Time: 15 Minutes

Ingredients:

- 1 cup canned pumpkin (no salt added)
- 1/2 cup low-fat vanilla yogurt
- 2 tablespoons brown sugar
- 1/2 teaspoon ground cinnamon
- 1/4 teaspoon ground nutmeg
- 1/4 teaspoon ground ginger

Cooking Instructions:

1. In a bowl, combine canned pumpkin, low-fat vanilla yogurt, brown sugar, ground cinnamon, ground nutmeg, and ground ginger.
2. Mix until smooth and refrigerate for at least 30 minutes.

Nutritional Information (per serving): Approximately 70 calories, 2g protein, 16g carbohydrates, 3g fiber, 9g sugar, 0g fat, 20mg sodium.

Modification Tip: For lower sodium, use a salt substitute. To reduce potassium, consume a smaller portion.

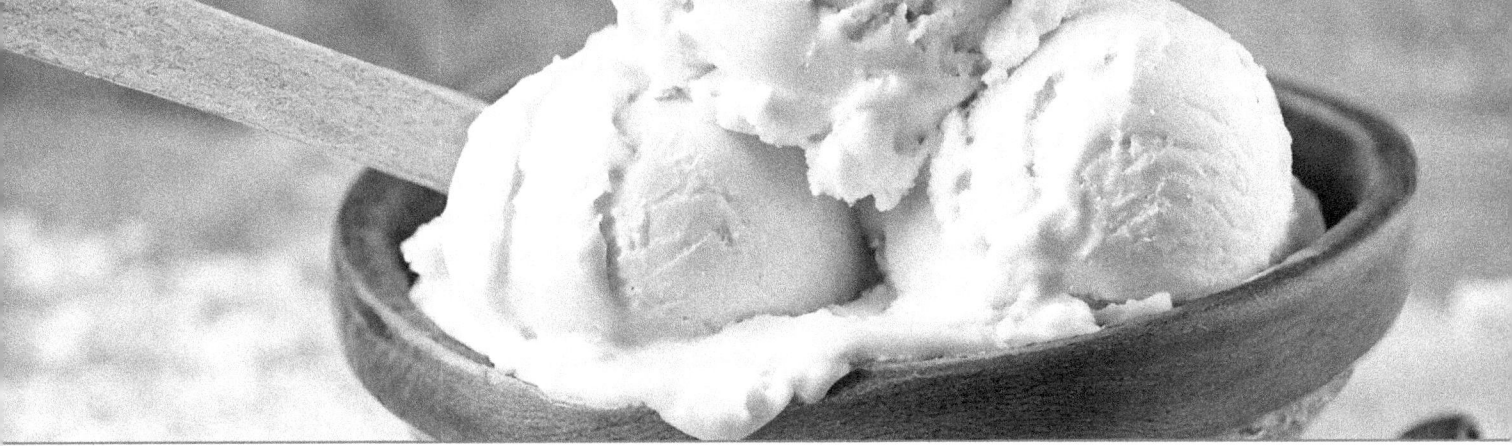

53. Banana Ice Cream

Benefits: This dessert offers a taste of pumpkin pie without the high potassium and phosphorus content.

Servings: 2

Prep/Cook Time: 10 Minutes

Ingredients:

- 2 ripe bananas
- 1/4 cup low-fat milk
- 1 teaspoon vanilla extract
- 1/4 teaspoon ground cinnamon

Cooking Instructions:

1. Slice the ripe bananas and freeze them for at least 2 hours.
2. In a blender or food processor, combine frozen banana slices, low-fat milk, vanilla extract, and ground cinnamon.
3. Blend until you achieve a creamy ice cream consistency.

Nutritional Information (per serving): Approximately 100 calories, 2g protein, 24g carbohydrates, 3g fiber, 12g sugar, 0g fat, 20mg sodium.

Modification Tip: For lower sodium, use a salt substitute. To reduce potassium, consume a smaller portion.

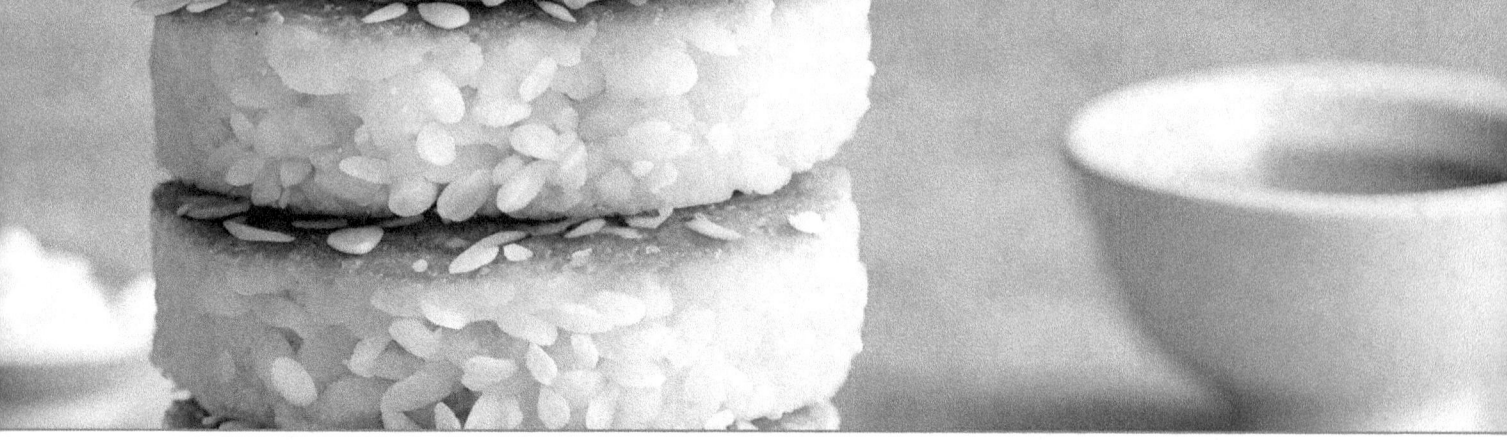

54. Almond Rice Cakes

Benefits: These almond rice cakes provide a sweet and crunchy snack without excess potassium or phosphorus.

Servings: 2

Prep/Cook Time: 5 Minutes

Ingredients:

- 2 rice cakes
- 2 tablespoons almond butter
- 1/2 banana, sliced
- 1/2 teaspoon honey (optional)

Cooking Instructions:

1. Spread almond butter on the rice cakes.
2. Top with banana slices and drizzle with honey if desired.

Nutritional Information (per serving): Approximately 160 calories, 4g protein, 22g carbohydrates, 2g fiber, 8g sugar, 7g fat, 0mg sodium.

Modification Tip: For lower sodium, use a salt substitute. To reduce potassium, consume a smaller portion of banana.

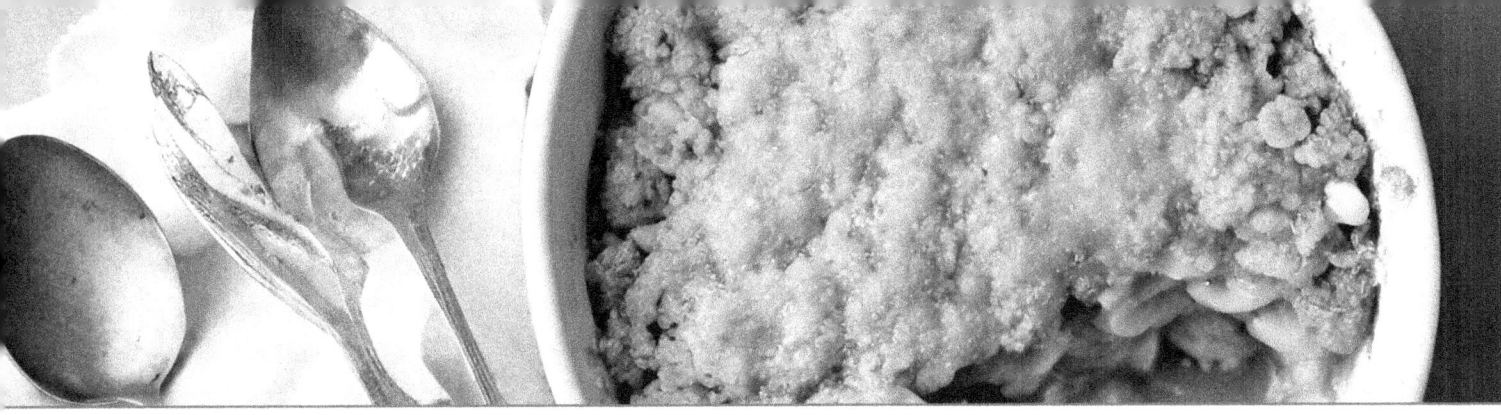

55. Apple Crisp

Benefits: This apple crisp is a warm and comforting dessert that's low in potassium and phosphorus.

Servings: 4

Prep/Cook Time: 45 Minutes

Ingredients:

- 4 cups apples, peeled and sliced
- 1/2 cup old-fashioned oats
- 1/4 cup all-purpose flour
- 1/4 cup brown sugar
- 1/4 cup unsalted butter
- 1/2 teaspoon ground cinnamon

Cooking Instructions:

1. Preheat the oven to 350°F (175°C).
2. In a baking dish, place peeled and sliced apples.
3. In a bowl, combine old-fashioned oats, all-purpose flour, brown sugar, unsalted butter (cut into small pieces), and ground cinnamon.
4. Mix until it resembles coarse crumbs.
5. Sprinkle the oat mixture evenly over the apples.
6. Bake for about 30-35 minutes, or until the topping is golden brown and the apples are tender.

Nutritional Information (per serving): Approximately 250 calories, 2g protein, 45g carbohydrates, 4g fiber, 26g sugar, 10g fat, 0mg sodium.

Modification Tip: For lower sodium, use a salt substitute. To reduce potassium, consume a smaller portion.

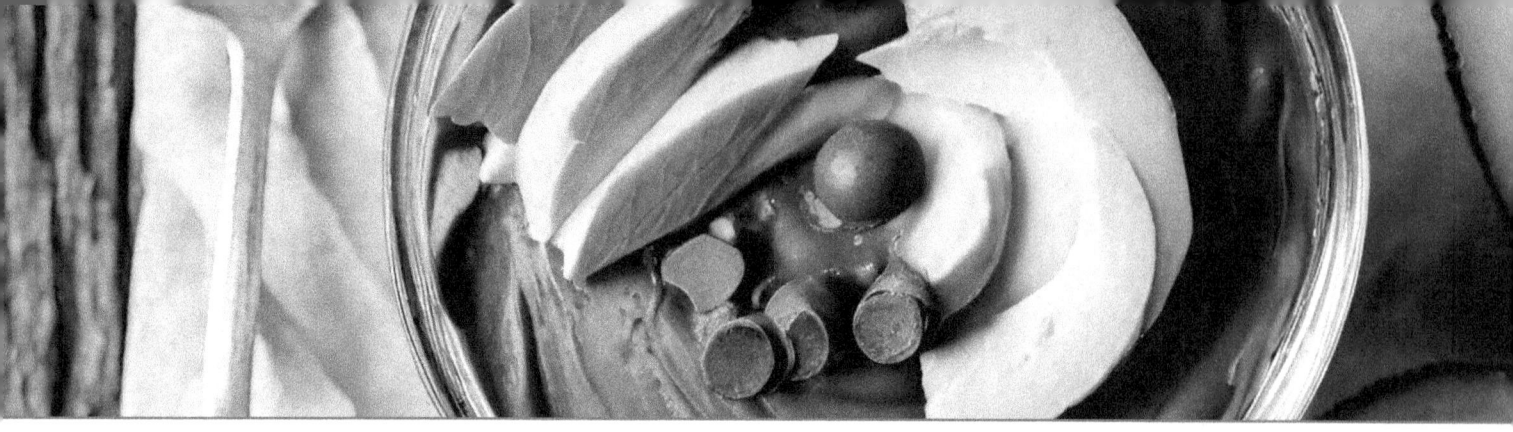

56. Chocolate Avocado Pudding

Benefits: This pudding is a creamy and chocolaty treat with reduced potassium and phosphorus.

Servings: 2

Ingredients:

- 1 ripe avocado
- 1/4 cup unsweetened cocoa powder
- 1/4 cup honey (or a sugar substitute)
- 1/4 cup low-fat milk
- 1/2 teaspoon vanilla extract

Prep/Cook Time: 10 Minutes

Cooking Instructions:

1. Scoop the flesh of a ripe avocado into a blender or food processor.
2. Add unsweetened cocoa powder, honey (or sugar substitute), low-fat milk, and vanilla extract.
3. Blend until smooth.
4. Refrigerate for at least 30 minutes before serving.

Nutritional Information (per serving): Approximately 240 calories, 3g protein, 35g carbohydrates, 6g fiber, 24g sugar, 13g fat, 20mg sodium.

Modification Tip: For lower sodium, use a salt substitute. To reduce potassium, consume a smaller portion.

57. Lemon Sorbet

Benefits: This lemon sorbet is a refreshing and tangy dessert that's low in potassium and phosphorus.

Servings: 4

Prep/Cook Time: 10 Minutes

Ingredients:

- 1 cup lemon juice
- 1 cup water
- 1/2 cup granulated sugar
- Zest of 1 lemon

Cooking Instructions:

1. In a saucepan, combine water, granulated sugar, and lemon zest. Heat over low heat, stirring until the sugar is dissolved.
2. Remove from heat and let the syrup cool.
3. In a bowl, mix lemon juice and the cooled syrup.
4. Pour the mixture into an ice cream maker and churn according to the manufacturer's instructions.
5. Transfer to a container and freeze for a few hours until firm.

Nutritional Information (per serving): Approximately 100 calories, 0g protein, 26g carbohydrates, 0g fiber, 24g sugar, 0g fat, 0mg sodium.

Modification Tip: For lower sodium, use a salt substitute. To reduce potassium, consume a smaller portion.

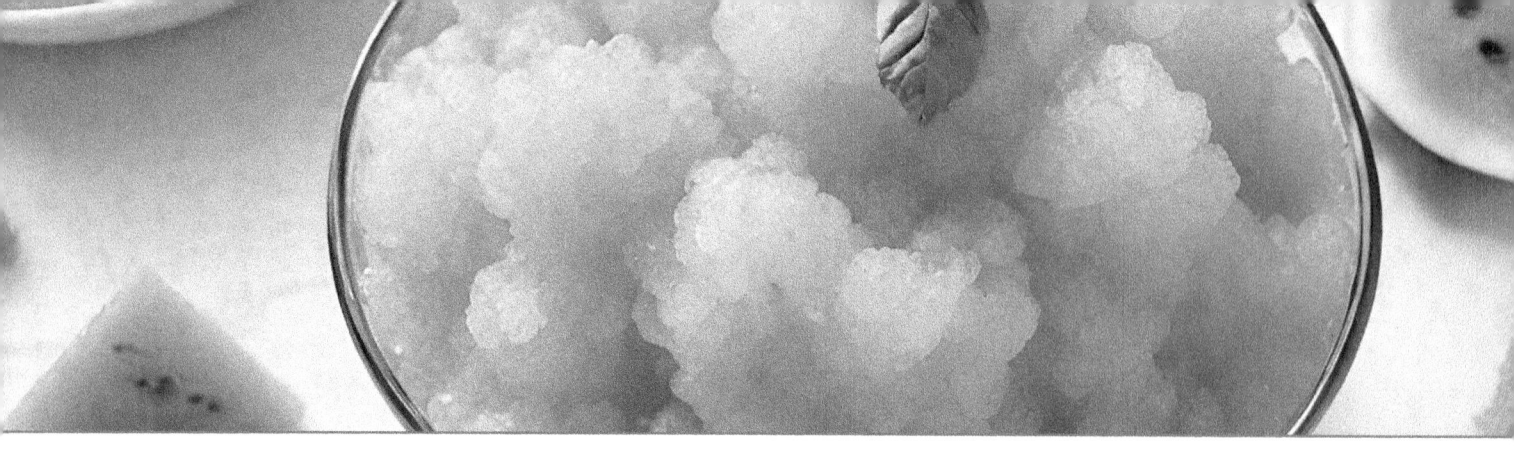

58. Watermelon Granita

Benefits: This watermelon granita is a cooling and low-potassium dessert option.

Servings: 4

Prep/Cook Time: 10 Minutes

Ingredients:

- 4 cups seedless watermelon, cubed
- 1/4 cup granulated sugar
- Juice of 1 lime

Cooking Instructions:

1. Place cubed watermelon in a blender and puree until smooth.
2. In a bowl, combine watermelon puree, granulated sugar, and lime juice.
3. Pour the mixture into a shallow dish and place it in the freezer.
4. Every 30 minutes, scrape the mixture with a fork to create a granita texture. Repeat this process for 2-3 hours or until the granita is fully frozen.

Nutritional Information (per serving): Approximately 90 calories, 1g protein, 23g carbohydrates, 0g fiber, 22g sugar, 0g fat, 0mg sodium.

Modification Tip: For lower sodium, use a salt substitute. To reduce potassium, consume a smaller portion.

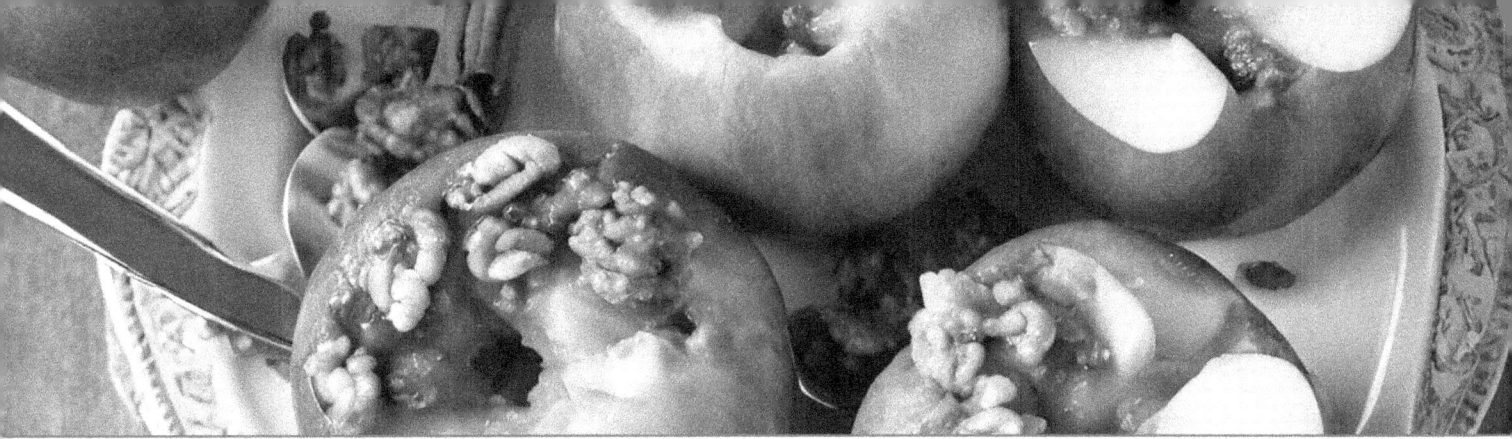

59. Baked Apples with Cinnamon and Walnuts

Benefits: This dessert is warm, comforting, and low in potassium and phosphorus.

Servings: 4

Prep/Cook Time: 40 Minutes

Ingredients:

- 4 medium-sized apples (such as Granny Smith)
- 1/4 cup chopped walnuts
- 1/4 cup brown sugar
- 1 teaspoon ground cinnamon
- 2 tablespoons unsalted butter (optional)

Cooking Instructions:

1. Preheat your oven to 350°F (175°C).
2. Wash the apples, and then core and hollow them, leaving the bottom intact. You can use an apple corer or a small knife.
3. In a bowl, combine chopped walnuts, brown sugar, and ground cinnamon. Optionally, add the unsalted butter to the mixture to create a richer filling.
4. Stuff each apple with the walnut mixture.
5. Place the stuffed apples in a baking dish and cover them with aluminum foil.

Cooking Instructions:

6. Bake for about 30 minutes or until the apples are tender. To check for doneness, insert a fork or knife; it should glide in easily.
7. Once baked, serve the apples warm. Optionally, top each with a small scoop of low-fat vanilla ice cream.

Nutritional Information (per serving): Approximately 180 calories, 2g protein, 30g carbohydrates, 4g fiber, 22g sugar, 7g fat, 0mg sodium.

Modification Tip: For lower sodium, use a salt substitute and skip the ice cream. To reduce potassium, consume a smaller portion of the stuffed apples.

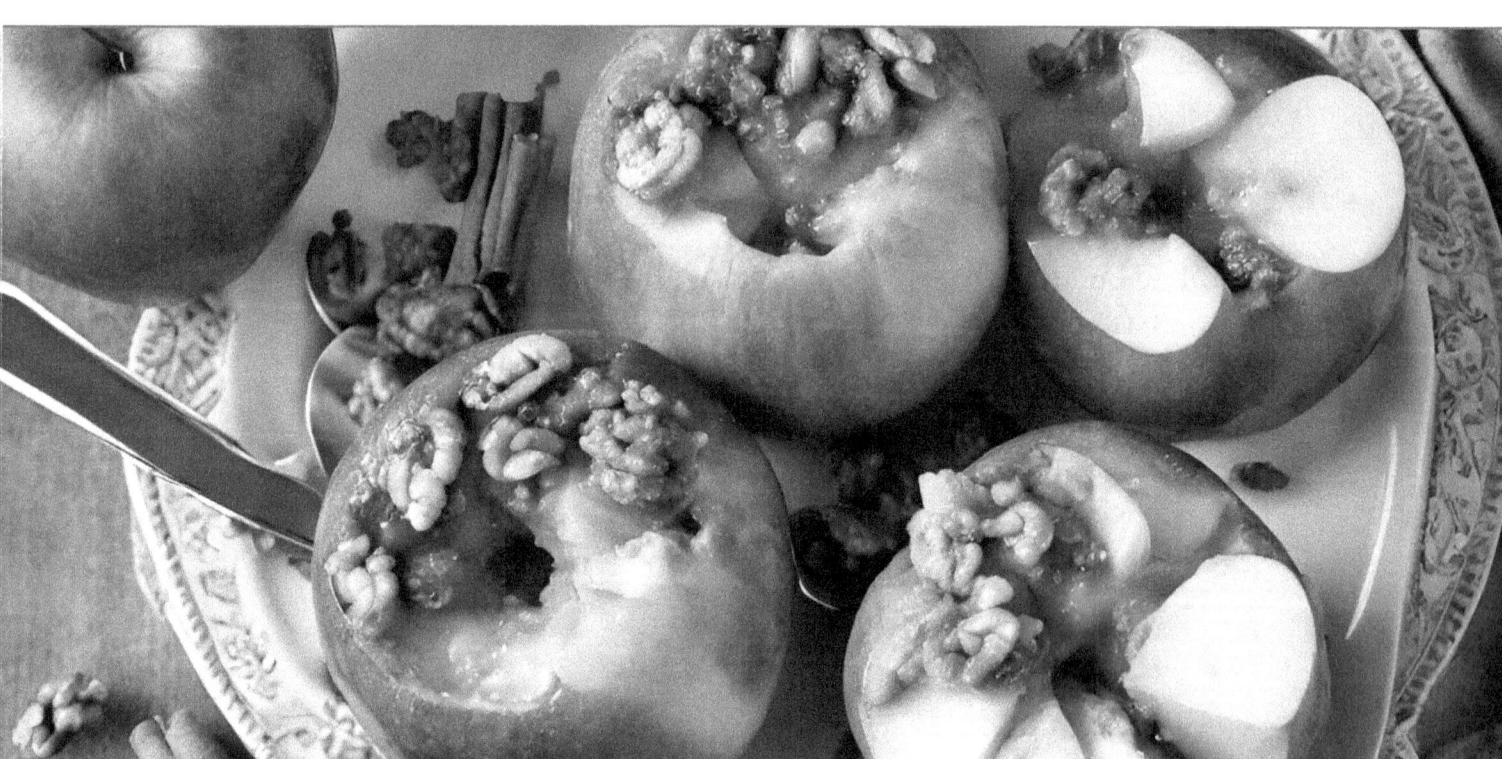

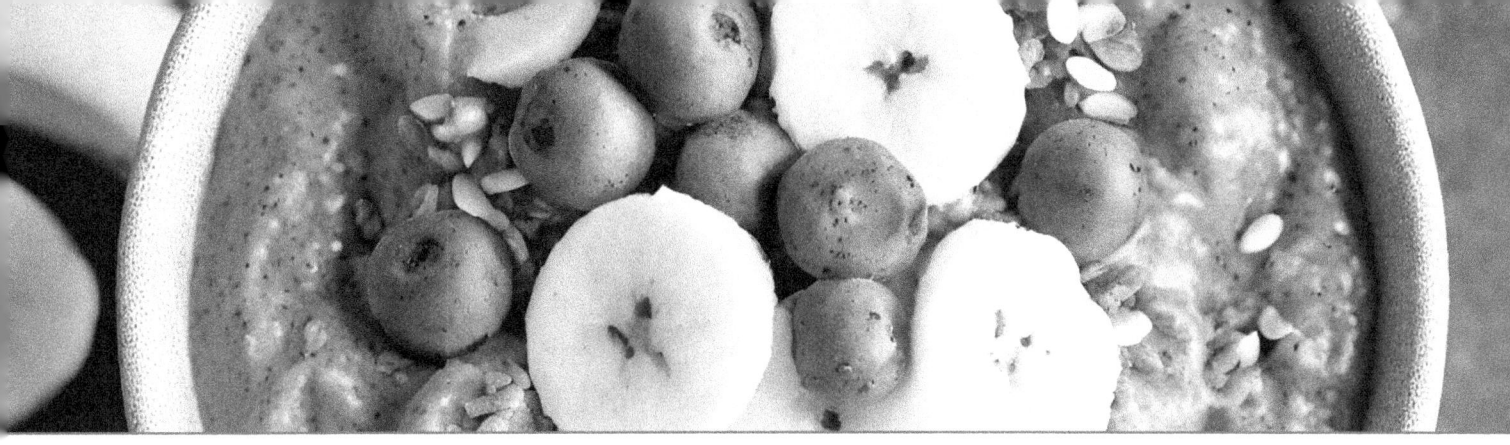

60. Chocolate Banana Chia Pudding

Benefits: This delightful dessert is perfect for satisfying your sweet cravings while supporting your kidney health.

Servings: 4

Ingredients:

- 2 ripe bananas, peeled and sliced
- 2 tablespoons unsweetened cocoa powder
- 2 tablespoons chia seeds
- 1/2 teaspoon vanilla extract
- 1 cup unsweetened almond milk
- 1-2 tablespoons honey or a sugar substitute (adjust to taste)
- Fresh berries or sliced bananas for garnish (optional)

Prep/Cook Time: 10 Minutes

Cooking Instructions:

1. In a blender, combine the ripe bananas, unsweetened cocoa powder, chia seeds, vanilla extract, and unsweetened almond milk.
2. Blend the mixture until it's smooth and well combined. If you prefer a sweeter taste, you can add honey or your preferred sugar substitute at this stage. Adjust the sweetness to your liking.
3. Once the pudding mixture is smooth, pour it into a bowl or individual serving glasses.
4. Cover the bowl or glasses with plastic wrap or lids and refrigerate for at least 4 hours or overnight. Chia seeds will absorb the liquid and create a thick, pudding-like texture.

5. When ready to serve, garnish with fresh berries or slices of banana if desired.

6. Enjoy your creamy, kidney-friendly chocolate banana chia pudding!

Nutritional Information (per serving): Approximately 170 calories, 3g protein, 32g carbohydrates, 8g fiber, 15g sugar, 6g fat, 335mg Potassium,.

Modification Tip:

- To reduce potassium, you can limit the amount of banana used or use a low-potassium fruit like pears.

- Adjust the sweetness level with honey, agave nectar, or a sugar substitute to accommodate your dietary preferences.

- For added texture, consider mixing in chopped nuts or seeds before refrigerating.

- Top with a dollop of low-phosphorus whipped cream or a sprinkle of crushed low-phosphorus cookies for an extra treat.

1.7 Cooking Techniques

Cooking techniques play a pivotal role in managing kidney disease, especially when it comes to controlling the intake of potassium and phosphorus. High levels of these minerals in the bloodstream can put added strain on the kidneys. By employing specific methods during food preparation, seniors can lower the potassium and phosphorus content in their meals.

One effective technique for reducing potassium in certain foods is soaking. Soaking high-potassium vegetables can help leach out some of the potassium, making them more kidney-friendly. Here's how this process works:

Soaking High-Potassium Vegetables: A Practical Approach

High-potassium vegetables such as potatoes, sweet potatoes, and winter squash are commonly used in a variety of dishes. While they offer excellent nutritional benefits, they can be problematic for individuals with kidney disease due to their elevated potassium content.

To reduce the potassium levels in these vegetables, the soaking technique can be employed:

1. **Peel and Slice:** Start by peeling and slicing the high-potassium vegetable into your desired shape or size. For example, if you're preparing potatoes for mashed potatoes, peel and slice them into cubes.
2. **Soaking:** Place the sliced vegetables in a large bowl of water. Ensure that the water completely covers the vegetable pieces. Soaking times can vary depending on the type of vegetable. For potatoes, a recommended soak time is at least two hours. During this time, potassium will leach out of the vegetable into the water.

3. **Rinse and Cook:** After the soaking period, drain the water from the vegetables and rinse them thoroughly under running water. This step helps to remove any excess potassium released during soaking.

4. **Cooking:** Now, the vegetables are ready to be cooked as desired. Boiling or steaming the soaked vegetables is a good choice, as these methods are known to reduce potassium content even further.

5. **Use of Excess Soak Water:** The water used for soaking can still contain potassium. Instead of discarding it, you can reuse this water for other purposes, such as watering plants or as a base for soups or stews, provided you monitor your overall daily potassium intake.

It's essential to note that while this technique can help reduce potassium levels in certain high-potassium vegetables, it may not completely eliminate potassium. Therefore, portion control remains crucial.

Boiling and Draining Technique

Boiling and draining is a straightforward and practical cooking technique that can help lower the potassium and phosphorus levels in various foods, making them more suitable for seniors with kidney disease. This method is particularly effective for high-potassium and high-phosphorus ingredients, such as beans, certain vegetables, and grains.

How to Boil and Drain for Potassium and Phosphorus Reduction:

1. **Prepare the Food:** Begin by washing and preparing the food item of your choice. This technique works well for dried beans, grains like rice, and certain vegetables such as spinach or collard greens.

2. Boil in Abundant Water: Place the food in a pot and cover it with a generous amount of water. For beans or grains, use several times the amount of water

compared to the food. Ensure there's enough water to keep the ingredients submerged throughout the cooking process.

3. **Boil Vigorously:** Bring the water to a vigorous boil and maintain this high heat for a specified time. The exact boiling time can vary depending on the food item. For beans, a good practice is to boil them for about 10 minutes.

4. **Drain and Rinse:** After the boiling process, carefully drain the boiling water from the food. This step is crucial as it removes a significant portion of the potassium and phosphorus that has leached out of the food during cooking. Rinse the food thoroughly under cold running water to further reduce these minerals.

5. **Continue Cooking:** If the food is not yet fully cooked, you can proceed with your chosen recipe, whether it's for a soup, stew, or another dish. The reduced potassium and phosphorus content will help make the meal more kidney-friendly.

Boiling and draining can be particularly effective for foods like beans and greens, which naturally contain higher levels of potassium and phosphorus. It's essential to note that while this technique helps, it may not eliminate all the potassium and phosphorus, so portion control remains important.

1.8 Grocery Shopping Guide For Kidney-Friendly Cooking

When following a kidney-friendly diet, making smart choices at the grocery store is essential. To simplify your shopping experience and ensure you have the right ingredients on hand, here is a comprehensive grocery shopping guide tailored to the recipes and principles outlined in this cookbook. **What to look for when you are in the grocery store:**

1. Fresh Vegetables:

1. Leafy Greens: Opt for low-potassium greens like kale, collard greens, or turnip greens.
2. Cauliflower: A versatile, low-potassium alternative to potatoes for mashing.
3. Bell Peppers: Colorful and low in potassium.
4. Cucumbers: Crisp and refreshing for salads.
5. Zucchini: A versatile, low-potassium option for roasting and grilling.
6. Tomatoes: Fresh and ripe for salads.
7. Onions and Garlic: Flavorful staples for savory dishes.
8. Carrots: Great for snacking or adding to recipes.

2. Lean Proteins:

1. Chicken: Skinless, boneless chicken breasts or thighs.
2. Turkey: Lean ground turkey or turkey breast.
3. Fish: Salmon, cod, or tilapia.
4. Tofu: For vegetarian or vegan recipes.
5. Eggs: A protein-rich breakfast option.

3. Grains and Legumes:

4. Dairy and Dairy Alternatives:

1. Quinoa: A versatile and protein-rich grain.
2. White Rice: Lower in phosphorus compared to brown rice.
3. Pasta: Choose white pasta, and be mindful of portion sizes.
4. White Bread: Lower in phosphorus than whole-grain options.
5. **Dried Beans:** Choose lower-potassium varieties like navy beans or pinto beans.

5. Fruits:

1. Apples: A low-potassium fruit for snacking.
2. Berries: Blueberries, strawberries, and raspberries.
3. Lemons: For adding flavor to dishes.
4. **Pears:** A low-potassium option for desserts**.**

7. Nuts and Nut Butters:

1. Low-Fat Milk: Choose low-fat cow's milk or a dairy-free alternative like almond milk.
2. Greek Yogurt: A great source of protein.
3. Cottage Cheese: Opt for low-sodium varieties.

6. Herbs and Spices:

1. Herbs: Fresh or dried herbs like basil, parsley, and thyme.
2. Spices: Ground spices like cinnamon, garlic powder, and black pepper.

8. Canned and Packaged Foods:

1. Almonds: A source of healthy fats and protein.
2. Peanut Butter: Opt for unsalted varieties.

1. Canned Tuna: A versatile, low-phosphorus protein source.
2. Low-Sodium Broth: For soups and stews.
3. Canned Beans: Look for low-sodium options.

9. Sweeteners:

1. Honey: For natural sweetness.
2. Sugar Substitutes: When necessary for reducing sugar content

10. Miscellaneous:

1. Cooking Oils: Olive oil or vegetable oil for cooking.
2. Vinegar: For salad dressings and marinades.
3. Low-Sodium Soy Sauce: A flavor enhancer for savory dishes.
4. Salt Substitute: If recommended by your healthcare provider.

Remember to check labels for potassium and phosphorus content, and opt for low-sodium or unsalted options whenever possible. Additionally, consider using fresh or frozen ingredients over canned or processed foods to have more control over your nutrient intake.

1.9 Portion Control

Portion control is a fundamental aspect of managing kidney disease and maintaining a kidney-friendly diet. For seniors in stage 3 kidney disease, carefully monitoring the amount of food consumed is crucial to avoid overloading the body with excess nutrients like potassium and phosphorus, which the kidneys may struggle to process. Here are some essential guidelines for portion control:

1. **Know Your Serving Sizes:** Familiarize yourself with standard serving sizes for different food groups. Use measuring cups, scales, and portion control tools to help you accurately gauge portion sizes.

2. **Adjust for Your Needs:** Understand that everyone's dietary requirements are unique. Adjust your portion sizes based on your individual dietary restrictions, as recommended by your healthcare provider or dietitian.

3. **Use Smaller Plates:** Opt for smaller plates and bowls. This can create the illusion of a full plate and help control portion sizes.

4. **Mindful Eating:** Slow down and savor each bite. Pay attention to your body's hunger and fullness cues. This helps prevent overeating.

5. **Split Large Portions:** When dining out, sharing a meal with a friend or asking for a to-go container immediately can help control portions. Many restaurant servings are larger than necessary.

6. **Pre-Portion Snacks:** Instead of eating snacks directly from the package, divide them into single servings to prevent mindless munching.

7. **Control Portions of High-Potassium Foods:** Pay special attention to high-potassium foods like bananas or potatoes. Even kidney-friendly foods should be consumed in moderation.

8. **Limit High-Phosphorus Foods:** Similarly, control portion sizes for high-phosphorus foods like dairy products. Choose low-phosphorus alternatives when possible.

9. **Monitor Protein Intake:** While protein is essential, excessive protein intake can strain the kidneys. Measure and control your protein portions.

2.0 Tips For Dining Out

Dining out can be enjoyable, even when following a kidney-friendly diet. Here are some tips to make your restaurant experience healthier:

1. **Research Ahead:** Look up the menu online and choose kidney-friendly options before you arrive.

2. **Ask Questions:** Don't hesitate to ask your server about ingredient substitutions, portion sizes, or preparation methods.

3. **Request Customization:** Many restaurants are willing to adjust dishes to meet your dietary needs. For instance, you can ask for sauces on the side or have vegetables steamed instead of fried.

4. **Share or Box Half:** Split an entrée with a dining companion, or ask for a to-go box to take half the meal home before you even start eating.

5. **Beware of High-Sodium Options:** Restaurant dishes often contain high levels of sodium. Choose options with reduced salt when possible.

6. **Avoid All-You-Can-Eat:** Steer clear of all-you-can-eat buffets or deals, as they can lead to overeating.

7. **Stay Hydrated:** Drink water throughout the meal to help control your appetite and prevent excessive eating.

8. **Skip Desserts:** Consider forgoing dessert, or opt for a simple, low-phosphorus, and low-potassium choice like sorbet.

9. **Be Prepared:** Carry snacks or a meal replacement if you're unsure of the available options when dining out.

10. **Speak Up:** Inform your dining companions about your dietary restrictions to reduce pressure to overindulge.

By practicing portion control and following these tips when dining out, you can maintain your kidney-friendly diet while still enjoying restaurant meals. Remember that consistent communication with your healthcare provider or dietitian is crucial for personalized guidance and adjustments to your diet based on your specific needs and progress.

CHAPTER TWO: 30-DAY KIDNEY-FRIENDLY MEAL PLAN

WEEK 1

DAY	BREAKFAST	LUNCH	DINNER	SNACK
1	Scrambled Egg Whites with Spinach	Lemon-Herb Grilled Chicken	Grilled Lemon Herb Shrimp	Cottage Cheese with Berries
2	Banana and Almond Butter Pancakes	Quinoa and Vegetable Salad	Baked Cod with Roasted Vegetables	Baked Sweet Potato Fries
3	Avocado and Tomato Toast	Baked Salmon with Dill	Lemon and Herb Roasted Chicken	Greek Yogurt Parfait
4	Oatmeal with Fresh Berries	Black Bean and Vegetable Soup	Vegetable and Lentil Stir-Fry	Hummus with Cucumber Slices
5	Greek Yogurt Parfait	Turkey and Cranberry Wrap	Stuffed Bell Peppers with Ground Turkey	Rice Cake with Almond Butter
6	Apple-Cinnamon Rice Pudding	Cucumber and Dill Salad	Herbed Quinoa with Roasted Vegetables	Mixed Nuts
7	Spinach and Mushroom Frittata	Vegetable Stir-Fry with Tofu	Sweet Potato and Chickpea Curry	Celery and Cream Cheese

WEEK 2

DAY	BREAKFAST	LUNCH	DINNER	SNACK
8	Cottage Cheese with Pineapple	Egg Salad with Fresh Herbs	Lemon and Garlic Baked Tilapia	Sliced Apples with Peanut Butter
9	Blueberry-Banana Smoothie	Lentil Soup	Ratatouille	Carrot Sticks with Guacamole
10	Hummus with Cucumber Slices	Quinoa and Vegetable Salad	Baked Cod with Roasted Vegetables	Baked Sweet Potato Fries

11	Avocado and Tomato Toast	Baked Salmon with Dill	Lemon and Herb Roasted Chicken	Greek Yogurt Parfait
12	Oatmeal with Fresh Berries	Black Bean and Vegetable Soup	Vegetable and Lentil Stir-Fry	Hummus with Cucumber Slices
13	Scrambled Egg Whites with Spinach	Lemon-Herb Grilled Chicken	Grilled Lemon Herb Shrimp	Cottage Cheese with Berries
14	Greek Yogurt Parfait	Turkey and Cranberry Wrap	Stuffed Bell Peppers with Ground Turkey	Rice Cake with Almond Butter

WEEK 3

15	Cottage Cheese with Pineapple	Egg Salad with Fresh Herbs	Lemon and Garlic Baked Tilapia	Sliced Apples with Peanut Butter
16	Blueberry-Banana Smoothie	Lentil Soup	Ratatouille	Carrot Sticks with Guacamole
17	Scrambled Egg Whites with Spinach	Lemon-Herb Grilled Chicken	Grilled Lemon Herb Shrimp	Cottage Cheese with Berries
18	Banana and Almond Butter Pancakes	Quinoa and Vegetable Salad	Quinoa and Vegetable Salad	Baked Sweet Potato Fries
19	Avocado and Tomato Toast	Baked Salmon with Dill	Lemon and Herb Roasted Chicken	Greek Yogurt Parfait
20	Oatmeal with Fresh Berries	Black Bean and Vegetable Soup	Vegetable and Lentil Stir-Fry	Hummus with Cucumber Slices
21	Greek Yogurt Parfait	Turkey and Cranberry Wrap	Stuffed Bell Peppers with Ground Turkey	Rice Cake with Almond Butter

WEEK 3

22	Banana and Almond Butter Pancakes	Quinoa and Vegetable Salad	Baked Cod with Roasted Vegetables	Baked Sweet Potato Fries

23	Greek Yogurt Parfait	Turkey and Cranberry Wrap	Stuffed Bell Peppers with Ground Turkey	Rice Cake with Almond Butter
24	Scrambled Egg Whites with Spinach	Lemon-Herb Grilled Chicken	Grilled Lemon Herb Shrimp	Cottage Cheese with Berries
25	Spinach and Mushroom Frittata	Vegetable Stir-Fry with Tofu	Sweet Potato and Chickpea Curry	Celery and Cream Cheese
26	Avocado and Tomato Toast	Baked Salmon with Dill	Lemon and Herb Roasted Chicken	Greek Yogurt Parfait
27	Apple-Cinnamon Rice Pudding	Cucumber and Dill Salad	Herbed Quinoa with Roasted Vegetables	Mixed Nuts
28	Oatmeal with Fresh Berries	Black Bean and Vegetable Soup	Vegetable and Lentil Stir-Fry	Hummus with Cucumber Slices
29	Hummus with Cucumber Slices	Quinoa and Vegetable Salad	Baked Cod with Roasted Vegetables	Baked Sweet Potato Fries
30	Scrambled Egg Whites with Spinach	Lemon-Herb Grilled Chicken	Grilled Lemon Herb Shrimp	Cottage Cheese with Berries

CONCLUSION

In the journey of life, our health and well-being are precious companions, and as we age, they become even more paramount. For seniors, the challenges posed by chronic kidney disease in stage 3 can be daunting, but this cookbook has been crafted as a beacon of hope and empowerment. Throughout these pages, we have delved into the intricate realm of kidney health, recognizing the growing prevalence of this condition among our senior population and the imperative role that diet plays in its management.

As we conclude this culinary voyage through the world of kidney-friendly cuisine, we do so with the unwavering belief that a well-informed and purposeful approach to nutrition can be a transformative force. The Kidney Disease Diet for Seniors on Stage 3 is not merely a compilation of recipes; it is a dedicated ally for seniors and their caregivers on the path to better health.

Our exploration began with an understanding of kidney disease, its stages, and the myriad factors contributing to its emergence. We delved into the prevalence of this condition in the elderly, recognizing that knowledge is power in the battle against it.

The cookbook has bridged the gap between health-conscious eating and culinary delight, showcasing that kidney-friendly food can be delectable, satisfying, and wholesome. Each recipe has been thoughtfully developed to harmonize with the dietary guidelines imperative for kidney health, striking the delicate balance between nutrition and flavor.

Through the pages of this cookbook, we've unlocked the secrets of portion control, enabling seniors to take charge of their nutritional intake. The art of mindful dining and grocery shopping has been demystified, making the practical aspects of maintaining a kidney-friendly diet accessible to all.

As we part ways with this cookbook, we hope it has ignited a spark of inspiration in the hearts of seniors and their loved ones. May its recipes infuse kitchens with warmth and health, and its knowledge pave the way to better living.

Thank You for Reading

We extend our heartfelt gratitude for choosing to explore our "Kidney Disease Diet for Seniors on Stage 3" cookbook. It's been our pleasure to be your culinary companion on this journey toward better health and well-being.

We hope the recipes, guidelines, and insights within these pages have proven both informative and delectable. Our mission is to empower you or your loved ones with the knowledge and resources necessary to make informed dietary choices while managing stage 3 kidney disease.

Your commitment to embracing a kidney-friendly diet is a testament to your dedication to health and vitality. Remember, you have the power to nurture your well-being with each mindful choice you make.

Should you ever find yourself in need of further guidance or inspiration, know that we are here to serve as your trusty companion, ready to rekindle your love for food while prioritizing your kidney health. Reach out to us via our active email address consultemilywilson@gmail.com.

Once again, thank you for your readership and trust in our culinary expertise. May your journey be filled with flavor, nourishment, and the renewal of health.

With warmest regards,

Dr. Emily M. Wilson

Health professional and Dietitian

KIDNEY DIET
Meal Planner

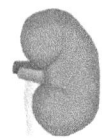

	BREAKFAST	LUNCH	DINNER
MON			
TUE			
WED			
THU			
FRI			
SAT			
SUN			

Your strength shines brightest in the face of adversity.
Keep shining; you are a beacon of hope

Date:
....

Shopping List

Note:

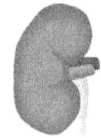 # KIDNEY DIET
Meal Planner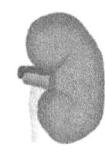

Date:
....

Shopping List

	BREAKFAST	LUNCH	DINNER
MON			
TUE			
WED			
THU			
FRI			
SAT			
SUN			

Your health is a reflection of the choices you make every day. Choose wisely, and you'll create a brighter future.

Note:

KIDNEY DIET
Meal Planner

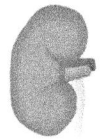 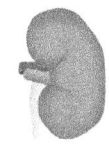

	BREAKFAST	LUNCH	DINNER
MON			
TUE			
WED			
THU			
FRI			
SAT			
SUN			

The path to healing begins with self-compassion. Be kind to yourself as you navigate this journey

Date:
....

Shopping List

Note:

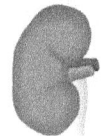 # KIDNEY DIET
Meal Planner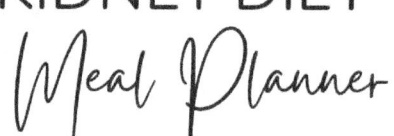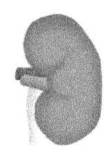

	BREAKFAST	LUNCH	DINNER
MON			
TUE			
WED			
THU			
FRI			
SAT			
SUN			

Patience is your greatest ally. Healing takes time, but every day brings you closer to your goals.

Date:

....

Shopping List

Note:

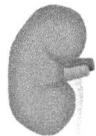# KIDNEY DIET
Meal Planner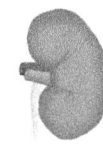

	BREAKFAST	LUNCH	DINNER
MON			
TUE			
WED			
THU			
FRI			
SAT			
SUN			

Surround yourself with positivity and people who believe
in your ability to overcome. Together, you are unstoppable

Date:
....

Shopping List

Note:

KIDNEY DIET
Meal Planner

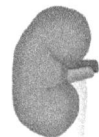 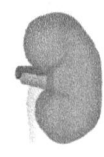

	BREAKFAST	LUNCH	DINNER
MON			
TUE			
WED			
THU			
FRI			
SAT			
SUN			

The journey to wellness may be long, but remember, you have the strength to make it.

Date:

....

Shopping List

Note:

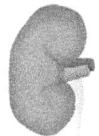 # KIDNEY DIET
Meal Planner
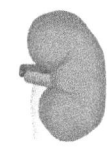

Date:
....

Shopping List

	BREAKFAST	LUNCH	DINNER
MON			
TUE			
WED			
THU			
FRI			
SAT			
SUN			

Hope is the heartbeat of resilience. Keep it alive, and you can conquer any obstacle.

Note:

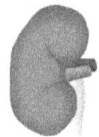# KIDNEY DIET
Meal Planner
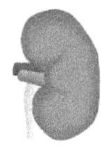

Date:

....

Shopping List

	BREAKFAST	LUNCH	DINNER
MON			
TUE			
WED			
THU			
FRI			
SAT			
SUN			

Your body is an incredible masterpiece. It has the power to heal and recover with the right care and love.

Note:

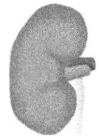 # KIDNEY DIET
Meal Planner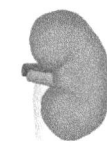

	BREAKFAST	LUNCH	DINNER
MON			
TUE			
WED			
THU			
FRI			
SAT			
SUN			

You are not defined by your diagnosis; you are defined by your courage and determination

Date:
....

Shopping List

Note:

KIDNEY DIET
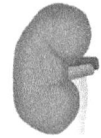 *Meal Planner*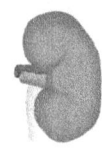

	BREAKFAST	LUNCH	DINNER
MON			
TUE			
WED			
THU			
FRI			
SAT			
SUN			

Small steps can lead to significant changes. Each healthy choice you make brings you closer to wellness.

Date:

....

Shopping List

Note:

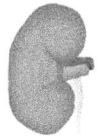 # KIDNEY DIET
Meal Planner
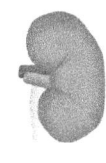

Date:

....

Shopping List

	BREAKFAST	LUNCH	DINNER
MON			
TUE			
WED			
THU			
FRI			
SAT			
SUN			

You are stronger than you know, and your spirit is more resilient than any challenge. Keep fighting, and never lose hope.

Note:

KIDNEY DIET
Meal Planner

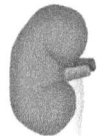 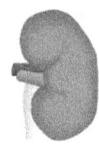

	BREAKFAST	LUNCH	DINNER
MON			
TUE			
WED			
THU			
FRI			
SAT			
SUN			

In the journey of life, challenges like kidney disease are just detours. Keep moving forward; your destination is worth the fight

Date:

....

Shopping List

Note:

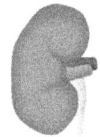 # KIDNEY DIET
Meal Planner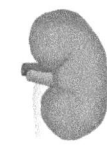

	BREAKFAST	LUNCH	DINNER
MON			
TUE			
WED			
THU			
FRI			
SAT			
SUN			

Your health is your most precious asset. Treat it with love, care, and the right nutrition.

Date:

....

Shopping List

Note:

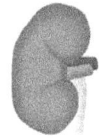 # KIDNEY DIET
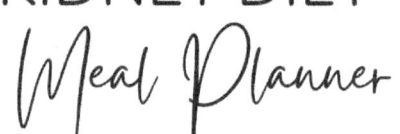
Meal Planner
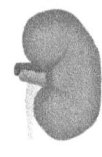

	BREAKFAST	LUNCH	DINNER
MON			
TUE			
WED			
THU			
FRI			
SAT			
SUN			

Believe in your inner strength; it's the fuel that keeps you going even when the road gets tough.

Date:
....

Shopping List

Note:

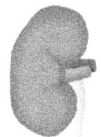 # KIDNEY DIET
Meal Planner
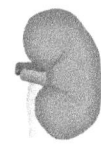

Date:

....

Shopping List

	BREAKFAST	LUNCH	DINNER
MON			
TUE			
WED			
THU			
FRI			
SAT			
SUN			

Every meal is a chance to nourish your body and nurture your kidneys. Embrace each bite as a step towards better health.

Note:

For an extra serving of kidney-friendly recipes, don't forget to peek at another delectable creation by the same author. It's like doubling down on deliciousness!

<u>SCAN THE QR CODE BELOW</u>

If you've got any burning questions about our tantalizing recipes or just want to chew the fat about your kidney health, drop me a line at my super-secret email hideout: consultemilywilson@gmail.com.

Oh, and by the way, reviews are the fuel that keeps this recipe train chugging along! If this cookbook has ignited your culinary passions and tamed your kidney woes, why not sprinkle a little review magic our way? It's the high-five of the internet world!

www.ingramcontent.com/pod-product-compliance
Lightning Source LLC
Chambersburg PA
CBHW082136290526
45794CB00008B/3058